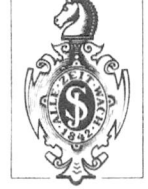

K. Hirohata M. Kurosaka T.D.V. Cooke (Eds.)

Joint Surgery
Up to Date

With 89 Figures

Springer Japan KK

KAZUSHI HIROHATA, MD
Professor and Chairman
Department of Orthopedics
Kobe University School of Medicine
Kobe, 650 Japan

MASAHIRO KUROSAKA, MD
Lecturer
Department of Orthopedics
Kobe University School of Medicine
Kobe, 650 Japan

T. DEREK V. COOKE, MA, MB, B Chir, FRCS(C)
Professor and Chairman
Clinical Mechanics Group
Queen's University
Kingston, Ontario
K7L 3NG Canada

ISBN 978-4-431-68098-7   ISBN 978-4-431-68096-3 (eBook)
DOI 10.1007/ 978-4-431-68096-3

Library of Congress Cataloging-in-Publication Data
Joint surgery up to date/K. Hirohata, M. Kurosaka, T.D.V. Cooke (eds.).   p.   cm.
Papers dervied from presentations at an international symposium, held on Nov 7,
1987 at the Kobe International Conferences Center, in celebration of the 10th
anniversary of Dr. Kazushi Hirohata's professorship in the Orthopedic Dept. of Kobe
University. Includes bibliographical references. ISBN 0-387-70048-X (U.S.)
1. Artificial hip joints—Congresses. 2. Artificial knee—Congresses.
3. Arthroplasty—Congresses. I. Hirohata, Kazushi. II. Kurosaka, M. (Masahiro),
1951- . III. Cooke, T.D.V. (T. Derek V.), 1938-   . [DNLM: 1. Hip Prosthesis—
congresses. 2. Joint Prosthesis—congresses. 3. Knee Prosthesis—congresses. WE 850/
J745 1987] RD549.J65 1989, 617.5'8059—dc20, DNLM/DLC, for Library of Congress

© Springer Japan 1989
Originally published by Springer-Verlag Tokyo in 1989

The use of registered names, trademarks, etc. in this publication does not imply,
even in the absence of a specific statement, that such names are exempt from the
relevant protective laws and regulations and therefore free for general use.

Product liability: The publisher can give no guarantee for information about
drug dosage and application thereof contained in this book. In every individual
case the respective user must check its accuracy by consulting other pharmaceu-
tical literature.

Typesetting: Koford Prints (Pte) Ltd., Singapore

Preface

Surgical management of joint problems has progressed drama-
tically in the past few years. Clearer understanding of the patho-
genesis of joint disorders and recent additions to our knowledge of
joint mechanics have made formerly unimagined procedures
possible. Moreover, tremendous advancement in implant technology offers us a wider variety of surgical procedures and a better
chance of obtaining satisfactory results. At the same time,
alternative bone-preserving procedures, such as osteotomy, in the
weight-bearing joints are still of great significance in selected
cases. In this context, it is clear that international collaboration
and coordination of scientific endeavours is crucial. Over the last
decade, thanks to the great assistance given by contributors to this
book, we have tried to coordinate our endeavors on the international level without being restricted to our own societies. Therefore, it was fitting that the symposium was held in an effort to
bring together experts in the field of joint surgery to share their
specialized knowledge. We hoped that the free interchange of
ideas would bring about an updated understanding and provide
knowledge essential to the treatment of joint disease.

KAZUSHI HIROHATA

Table of Contents

Part 2. Problem Case Presentation and Surgical Decision Making

List of Contributors

CHANDLER, HUGH P.

Ambulatory Care Center, Level 4
Massachusetts General Hospital
15 Parkman Street, Boston
MA 02114, USA

COOKE, T. DEREK V.

Clinical Mechanics Group
Queen's University
Kingston, Ontario
K7L 3N6 Canada

HIROHATA, KAZUSHI

Department of Orthopedics
Kobe University School of Medicine
5-1, Kusunoki-cho 7-chome
Kobe, 650 Japan

KAWAI, KAZUO

Department of Orthopedics
Kobe University School of Medicine
5-1, Kusunoki-cho 7-chome
Kobe, 650 Japan

KUMMER, BENNO

Direktor des Anatomischen Instituts
Universität zu Köln
Josef-Stelzmann Strasse 9
5000 Köln 41,
Federal Republic of Germany

KUROSAKA, MASAHIRO

Department of Orthopedics
Kobe University School of Medicine
5-1, Kusunoki-cho 7-chome
Kobe, 650 Japan

MANN, ROGER A.

Associate Clinical Professor
Department of Orthopedic Surgery
University of California School of Medicine
3000 Webster Street Suite 1200, Oakland
CA 94577, USA

MIZUNO, KOSAKU   Department of Orthopedics
                              Kobe University School of Medicine
                              5-1, Kusunoki-cho 7-chome
                              Kobe, 650 Japan

MURATSU, HIROTSUGU   Department of Orthopedics
                              Kobe University School of Medicine
                              5-1, Kusunoki-cho 7-chome
                              Kobe, 650 Japan

SHIBA, RYOICHI   Department of Orthopedics
                              Kobe University School of Medicine
                              5-1, Kusunoki-cho 7-chome
                              Kobe, 650 Japan

SHIMIZU, TOMIO   Department of Orthopedics
                              Kobe University School of Medicine
                              5-1, Kusunoki-cho 7-chome
                              Kobe, 650 Japan

STAUFFER, RICHARD N.   Mayo Medical School
                              Department of Orthopedic Surgery
                              Mayo Clinic
                              200 First Street, S.W. Rochester
                              MN 55905, USA

STULBERG, BERNARD N.   Department of Orthopedic Surgery
                              The Cleveland Clinic Foundation
                              9500 Euclid Avneue, Cleveland
                              OH 44106, USA

WILDE, ALAN H.   Department of Orthopedic Surgery
                              The Cleveland Clinic Foundation
                              9500 Euclid Avenue, Cleveland
                              OH 44106, USA

Introduction

This book deals with recent developments in joint surgery with special focus on the problems of weight-bearing joints. The following papers were derived from presentations by guest speakers and the Kobe University staff at the international symposium held on November 7th, 1987 at the Kobe International Conference Center. This symposium was held in celebration of the 10th anniversary of Dr. Kazushi Hirohata's professorship in the Orthopedic Department of Kobe University. The symposium was organized into two sections: the first as formal presentations followed by discussions, and the second as a series of case reports illustrating interesting problems of the lower extremities. Bringing together a number of experts in the field of implant arthroplasty and concentrating on the problems of loosening, revision, and new developments as they apply to joint replacement, this book provides updated information on joint surgery for every orthopedic surgeon.

Part 1
Recent Advances and Problems in Total Joint Replacement

Biomechanics of Endoprostheses of the Hip and Adaptive Reactions of the Bone

Benno Kummer[1]

Summary. Following the hypothesis of Pauwels [1–3], the bone adapts to its actual mechanical stress by densification and apposition of new material or by decalcification and resorption. Increasing stress stimulates bone formation; decreasing stress stimulates resorption. However, extreme magnitudes of stress may lead to paradoxical loss of bone substance. Implantation of an endoprosthesis changes the mechanical stress of the bone considerably. It must be expected, therefore, that the structure and distribution of the bone material will change remarkably. These changes can be visualized and quantified by the densitometry of X-ray pictures. For this purpose, 5-mm-thick cross-sectional slices were taken from anatomical specimens of femora with implanted endoprostheses. X-rays of these slices were analyzed by computer-aided densitometry. Bone condensation was found at the sites of stress concentration. More transparent areas, however, could be attributed to either extremely low or extremely high stresses. This loss of bone material is responsible for the loosening of endoprostheses. These phenomena are demonstrated on examples of cementless and cemented femoral endoprostheses.

Introduction

Almost 100 years ago, W. Roux (1895) [4] assumed that bone formation and resorption is related to mechanical stresses. He pointed out that pressure forces or pressure alternating with tension stimulates ossification and that the amount of newly formed bone depends on the magnitude of the stresses. Absence of stresses or stresses below a certain limit should lead to bone resorption. The same theory attributed the connective tissue to tensile stresses and cartilage to shear stresses. So each of the three support tissues was linked to a particular type of stress.

About 50 years later, F. Pauwels [2, 3] profoundly reformed this histogenetic theory. He demonstrated with convincing arguments that there are only two primary tissues of support: connective tissue and cartilage. Deformation, due to compression, tension, or shear, should stimulate the formation of collagen fibers; while hydrostatic pressure was responsible for the differentiation of the mesenchyme into cartilage (Fig. 1). Both collagenous tissue and cartilage would be transformed into bone if they were stressed without any macroscopic deformation. Bone appears in Pauwels' theory as a secondary tissue of support. However, once formed, bone reacts

---

[1] Institute of Anatomy, University of Cologne, Cologne, Federal Republic of Germany

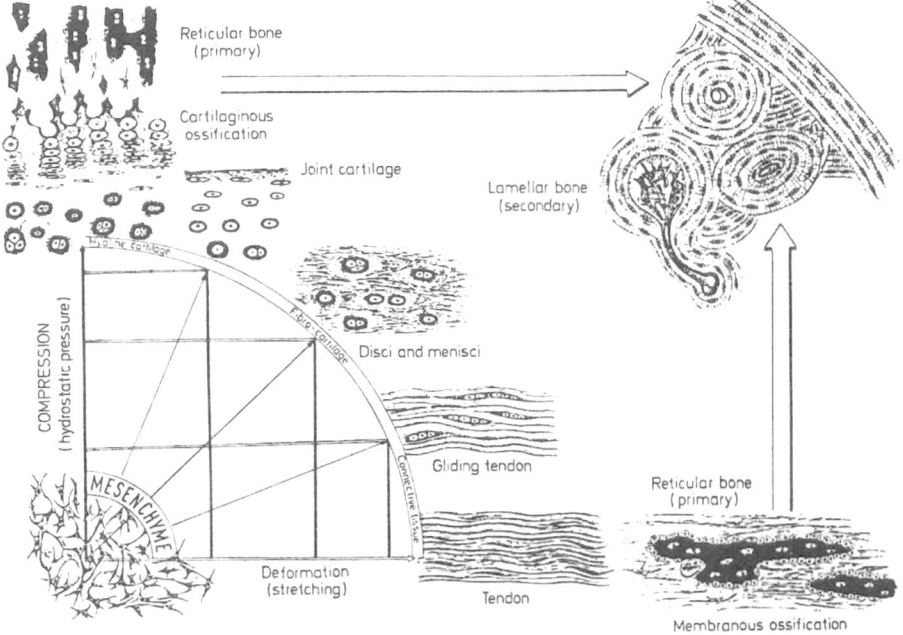

Fig. 1. Pauwels' hypothesis of casual histogenesis of the tissues of support shows pure hydrostatic pressure stimulates the differentiation of cartilage; pure tension is the specific stimulus for the formation of fibers. Intermediate tissues originate from combinations of hydrostatic pressure and tension. Bone is a secondary tissue of support, developing from cartilage as well as from connective tissue, and finally transforming into secondary lamellar bone

in a very characteristic manner to the actual stresses (independent of whether it is pressure, tension, or shear stress). An increase in stress stimulates bone formation; a decrease in stress causes a resorption response.

Bone Remodelling as a Feedback System

Therefore, bone may be regarded as a feedback system (Fig. 2). The final goal of this permanent remodelling is the approach to an equal distribution of stresses throughout the bone. Pauwels [1] published a mathematical model, demonstrating that only with the assumption of apposition or resorption in relation to the local stresses, a trabecular element of the spongy bone will finally be oriented exactly in the direction of the stressing force and it is therefore stressed by pure compression with equally distributed pressure stresses. Pauwels [2] showed furthermore that bone reacts to its actual stressing not only by remodelling in the sense of apposition and resorption of material but also by changing the local density of the tissue. Since these observations have been made from X-ray pictures, it is not truly clear whether the

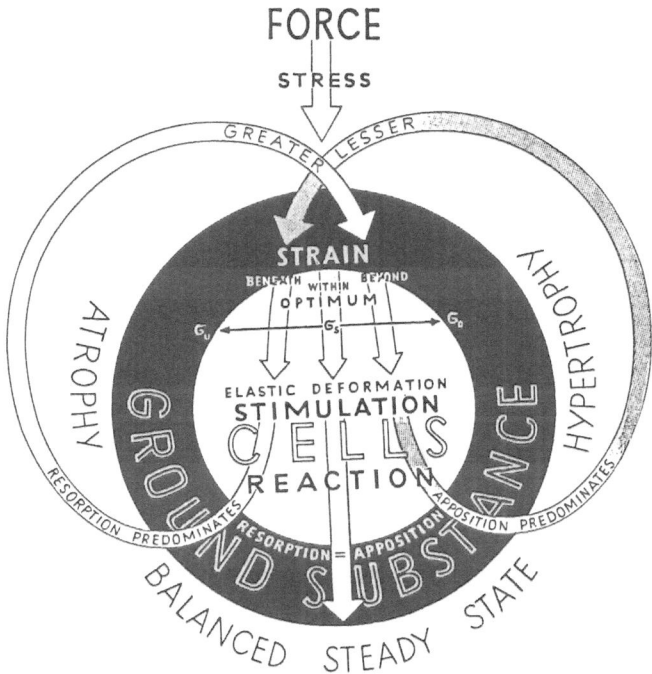

Fig. 2. Bone remodelling as a feedback system. The force causes micro-deformation (strain) that stimulates the cells (osteoblasts and osteoclasts). Only at a certain magnitude of strain the activities of osteoblasts and osteoclasts are balanced. Greater strain activates bone formation, lesser strain activates resorption

densification seen in the subchondral bone is due to increasing concentration of apatite or to the closure of porosities. The latter is at least one of the possible causes as can be demonstrated·in histological slices of densified bone. In the same publication [2], it was shown that overloading is followed by paradoxical bone resorption. Considering this, the apparition of the pseudo-cysts in osteoarthritic joints can be explained.

Mathematical Model of Pauwels' Hypothesis

Pauwels' hypothesis of bone remodelling can be expressed in mathematical terms (Fig. 3a). Based on this mathematical function, we developed a computer model of bone remodelling that fits very well to the observed transformations after pathological stressing. It shows very clearly, that in a tubular bone the thickness of the wall and the density of tissue increase at the sites where the stresses prior to the remodelling were greatest (Fig. 3b–e). We conclude from this, that the bone as a whole is

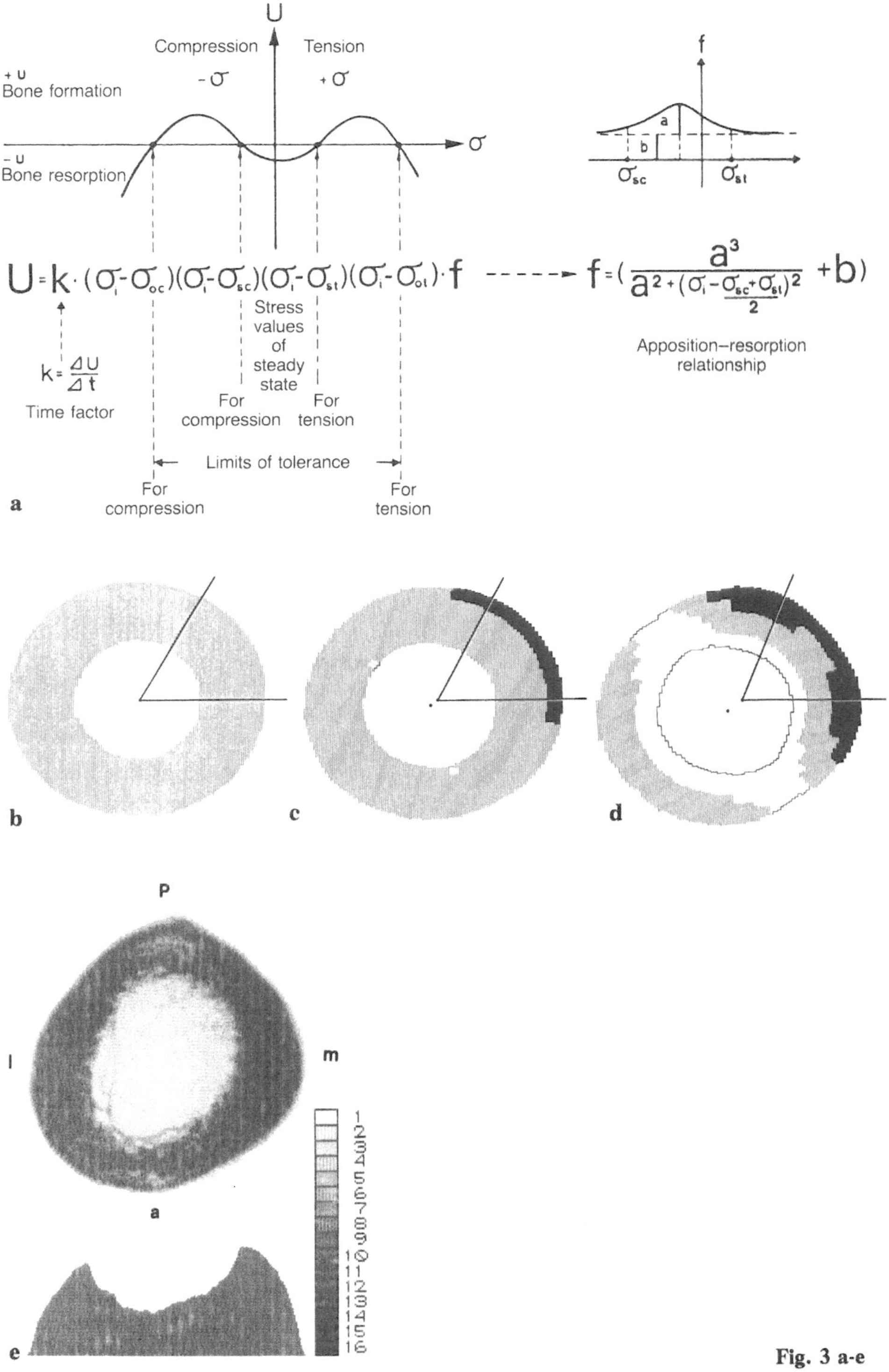

U

Compression   Tension

+ U
Bone formation $-\sigma$ $+\sigma$

σ

$-$ U
Bone resorption

f

a

b

σ_{sc} σ_{st}

$$U = k \cdot (\sigma_i - \sigma_{oc})(\sigma_i - \sigma_{sc})(\sigma_i - \sigma_{st})(\sigma_i - \sigma_{ot}) \cdot f \quad \dashrightarrow \quad f = \left(\frac{a^3}{a^2 + (\sigma_i - \frac{\sigma_{sc} + \sigma_{st}}{2})^2} + b \right)$$

Stress
values
of
steady
state

$k = \frac{\Delta U}{\Delta t}$

For   For
compression tension

Time factor

Apposition–resorption
relationship

Limits of tolerance

For   For
compression   tension

a

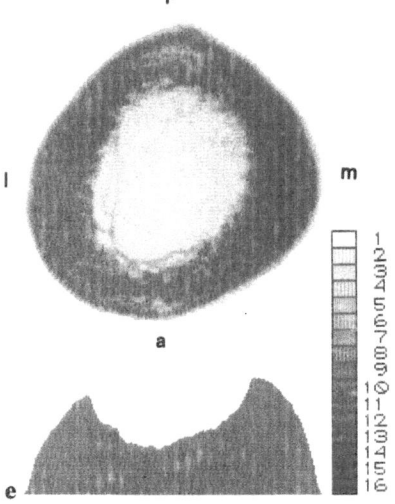

b   c   d

P

l   m

a

1
2
3
4
5
6
7
8
9
10
11
12
13
14
15
16

e

Fig. 3 a-e

under normal conditions, a well-adapted system with respect to its internal structure and the distribution of the dense material.

Removing parts of the bone and implanting an endoprosthesis decisively alters the direction and distribution of stresses and the process of remodelling starts, in which the local tissue reactions depend on the local quality and magnitude of stresses. Unfortunately we know this effect — mainly by the observations of Pauwels — only qualitatively. The exact values of the stresses which stimulate bone formation or destruction are still unknown. Nevertheless, the expected transformations of the bone would be predictable in principle if the actual stressing by the implant could be analyzed accurately.

The magnitude and direction of the hip resultant after implanting an endoprosthesis depend on the position of the center of rotation, total length and inclination of the neck and on the lever arm of the abductor muscles. It is rarely the case that all of these parameters remain the same. Therefore, different possibilities have to be considered. In general, the lever arm of the abductor muscles will more or less maintain its original length, and this is irregardless of whether the resected neck has been left long or short (Fig. 4). However, the muscular lever arm shortens remarkably if the neck of the prosthesis is placed in a more upright position.

Center of Rotation

The location of the center of rotation depends on the positions of the head and socket, the radius of the head and the thickness of the acetabular cup. The head of the prosthesis is in most types considerably smaller than the original femoral head. The center of the artificial joint therefore often lies more proximal (Fig. 4). The position of the articular center also depends on the shape of the acetabular cup, as has been previously mentioned. Shifting of the center of rotation along the neck axis alters the lever arms of the body weight and the muscle force, and consequently the

---

Fig. 3 a-e. Mathematical function, describing Pauwels' hypothesis on the functional adaptation of bone. **a** a and b factors, determining the relation between the magnitude of stresses and bone resorption; f, part of the function, influencing the bone resorption; k, factor, determining the speed of remodelling ("time factor"); σ, normal stresses; σ_i, actual stress; σ_{oc}, upper limit for compressive stresses; σ_{ot}, upper limit for tensile stresses; σ_{sc}, optimal compressive stress; σ_{st}, optimal tensile stress; t, time; U, rate of remodelling. **b** computer simulation of the functional adaptation of a tubular bone cross-section. Initial stage. The cross-section is exactly circular and the density is distributed uniformly. It is thought to be stressed by a pressure force, parallel to the bone's axis. The lever arm of the bending is indicated by the *black lines*. It is thought to change its direction in the angle between the two lines. They intersect at the inertial center of the cross-section. **c** After 6 steps of computer-simulated remodelling, the density in the bone changes. Higher density (at the pressure side of the bending) is represented by the *black* color, lowest density is marked by the *white* color. **d** After 72 steps of computer-simulated remodelling, the cross-section has changed its contour and density distribution remarkably. The steady state is reached and the "bone" is adapted to the imposed stress. **e** Densitometry of a cross-section of a tubular bone (femur). The *dark areas* represent sites of the highest density. The similarity to the "artificial bone" is obvious

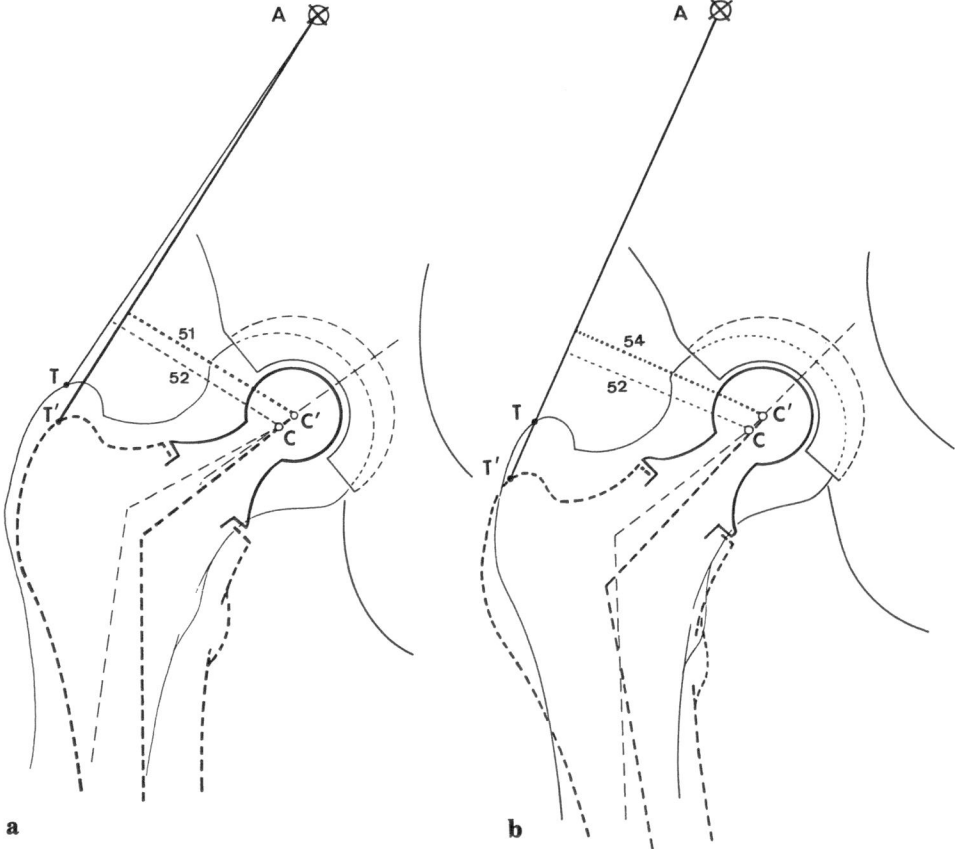

Fig. 4 a,b. Length of the lever arm of the abductor muscles of the hip. **a** in a femoral endoprosthesis with a relatively short stump of the neck. **b** in a prosthesis with a long neck stump. A, iliac insertion of abductors; C, center of the normal hip; C', center of rotation of the prosthesis; T, trochanteric insertion of abductors in the normal hip; T', trochanteric insertion in the hip with endoprosthesis. The numbers are the length of the lever arms (in mm)

resultant force changes its direction and magnitude (Fig. 5a). The total load on the joint increases with a distal shift of the center of rotation and decreases with a proximal shift, if the directions of body weight and muscle force vectors remain constant. Changing the direction of the muscle force vector means altering the lever arm of the muscle, and since the muscular moment must stay constant, the muscle force varies inversely with the lever arm length (Fig. 5b). Assumed that the point of intersection of muscle force and body weight vectors remains constant, the hip resultant force R maintains its direction, but changes in magnitude. The steeper the vector of the muscle force, the greater the resultant becomes.

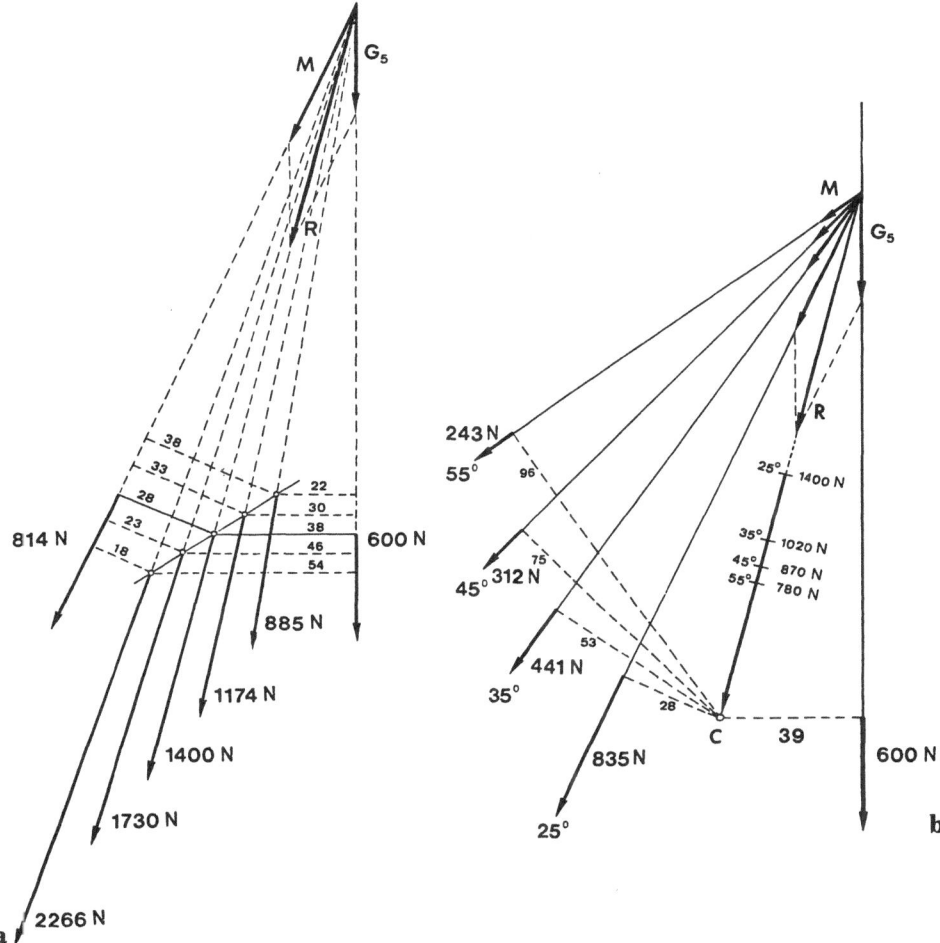

Fig. 5 a,b. Change of the direction and magnitude of the hip resultant in the position of the center of rotation. G_5, body weight; M, muscular force (abductors); R, hip resultant, small size numbers represent the lever arms of muscular forces and body weight (in mm), large size numbers give the forces in Newton. This model shows only theoretical relationship. The forces are relative values and do not represent the real values, since in reality the distance of the point of intersection of M and G_5 from the center of the hip joint is considerably longer. **b** Relationship between the direction of the muscular force and the magnitude of the hip resultant. Theoretical model. C, center of rotation; G_5, body weight; M, muscular force (abductors); R, hip resultant. For the different positions of the abductor force and different values of the resultant, the angle of inclination of muscle force against the vertical is indicated. Smaller numbers give the length of the lever arms (in mm)

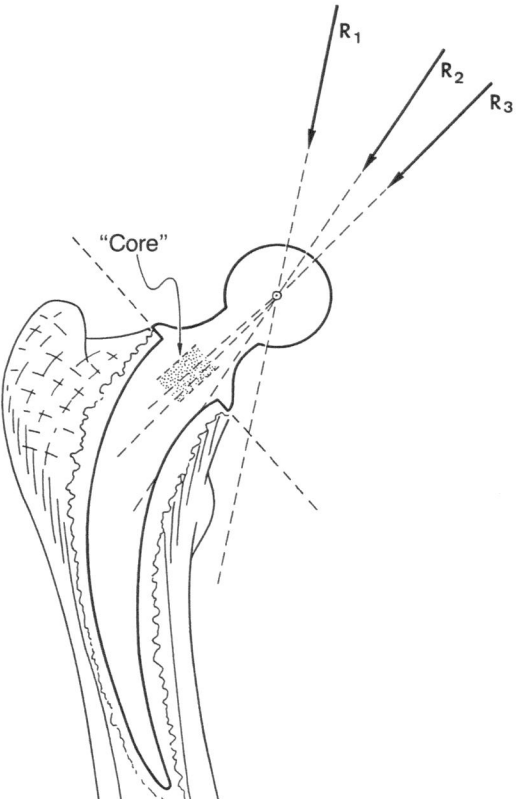

Fig. 6. Eccentricity of the hip resultant at the level of the collar of the prosthesis in relation to varying inclination of the resultant force. R_1, R_2, R_3, different positions of the resultant. There is pressure on the lateral side of the collar only if the line of action of the resultant lies inside the "core" of the prosthesis (R_3)

Stresses at the Bone-Cement Interface

However, in spite of all these changes in direction and magnitude of the joint resultant, the latter remains in any case more or less oblique to the neck axis, stressing the femoral neck by bending. For an implanted endoprosthesis, this eccentricity of the resultant force causes a tilting moment (Fig. 6). The force-transmission from the prosthesis to the bone depends on its anchorage. If both are firmly connected to each other by bone-cement, tensile forces can be transmitted. In this case, the bone-cement contact on the medial side is stressed by compression and the contact surface on the lateral side is stressed by tension. Since the main stress trajectories do not run exactly perpendicular to the bone-cement surface, shear stresses will occur, depending on the inclination of the main stresses with respect to the contact surface

(Fig. 7a, b). Theoretically this is true only for an even contact between bone and cement. In reality, the cement penetrates into the trabecular meshwork and therefore the force transmission is much more complex. Thus, along the entire interface, even at the sites of the main tensile stresses, pressure forces can be transmitted (Fig. 7c). These conclusions lead to the theoretical construction of a special type of a cementless prosthesis.

With or without cement, there are, in principle, two qualities of stresses to be transmitted between cement and bone: normal stresses (pressure or tension) and tangential stresses (shear). The latter can only be transmitted from one material to the other if they are "glued" together or if there is a sufficient coefficient of friction.

Following Pauwels' hypothesis of functional adaptation, the bone tissue will in both cases, either transmission of normal or tangential stresses, respond to the magnitude of stresses by apposition and densification or resorption and loss of calcium. In this regard, we will analyze two different cases of artificial hip replacement, obtained from the anatomical dissection course in Cologne. Radiographs were taken from the specimens with the prosthesis in situ, then 5-mm-thick transverse sections of bone and prosthesis were made. With the aid of a computer, charts of the density distribution were drawn from X-rays of the bone slices. By this method, the distribution of the material across the bone section can be analyzed.

Case Report

Case 1. The X-ray of the right femur of an 84-year-old woman shows densified bone at the medial wall of the neck stump, just beneath the collar of the prosthesis, and at the lateral wall of the diaphysis near the end of the prosthesis stem. Biomechanical analysis revealed that the densification appear precisely where the cementless implanted prosthesis presses against the bony wall (Fig. 8a). Since the hip resultant R is oriented oblique to the neck and the stem, the prosthesis is pivoting medially, supported at point A. Therefore, the end of the stem tends to move laterally and is resisted at point B.

Densitographs of transverse sections at levels A and B show that the dense zones in the X-ray of the total specimen are not the effects of projection, but specific points of condensation of the bone at the sites of maximal stress (Fig. 8b, c). With a new method, developed by my collaborator, M. Strauss (unpublished), the X-ray shadow of the metallic implant (and eventually of bone cement) can be eliminated by means of a computer program and the distribution of the bone material can be shown in a diagram.

Case 2. The second case concerns the femur of an 85-year-old woman with a cemented long-stem endoprosthesis (Fig. 9a). There, the bone in the region of the calcar is relatively transparent. Since the cement does not fill the medullar cavity till the end of the prosthesis stem, two versions of probable explanations must be discussed.

The first possible explanation is, that the prosthesis was more or less loose and tilted medially. If the pivot point were situated distally, then the prosthesis would press with a considerable momentum against the proximal medial wall and the bone

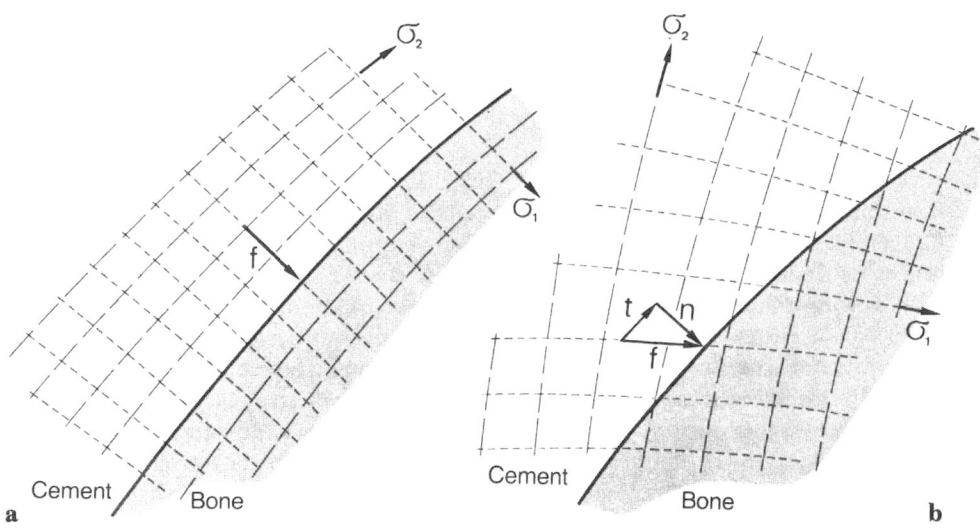

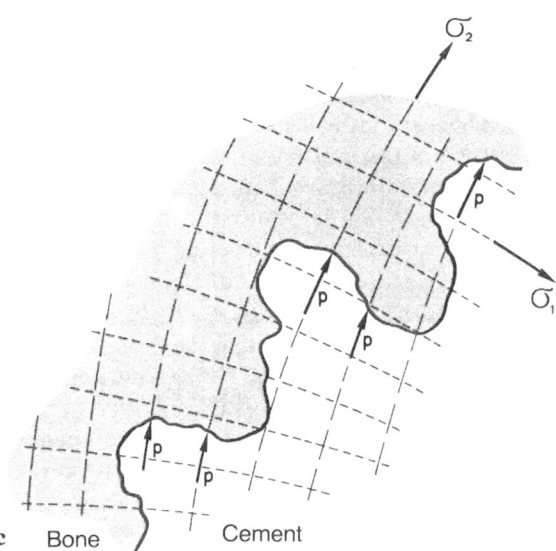

Fig. 7 a-c. Stresses at the bone-cement (or bone-implant) interface. **a** Compressive stresses are normal to the bone surface, no shear stresses occur. **b** The compressive stresses are oblique to the bone surface and tangential forces arise. f, original force; j_1, normal force; t, tangential force; σ_1, compressive stresses; σ_2, tensile stresses. **c** At the irregular boderline between the cement and bone, pressure forces are transmitted even at the site of main tensile stresses. p, pressure force; σ_1, main compressive stresses; σ_2, main tensile stress

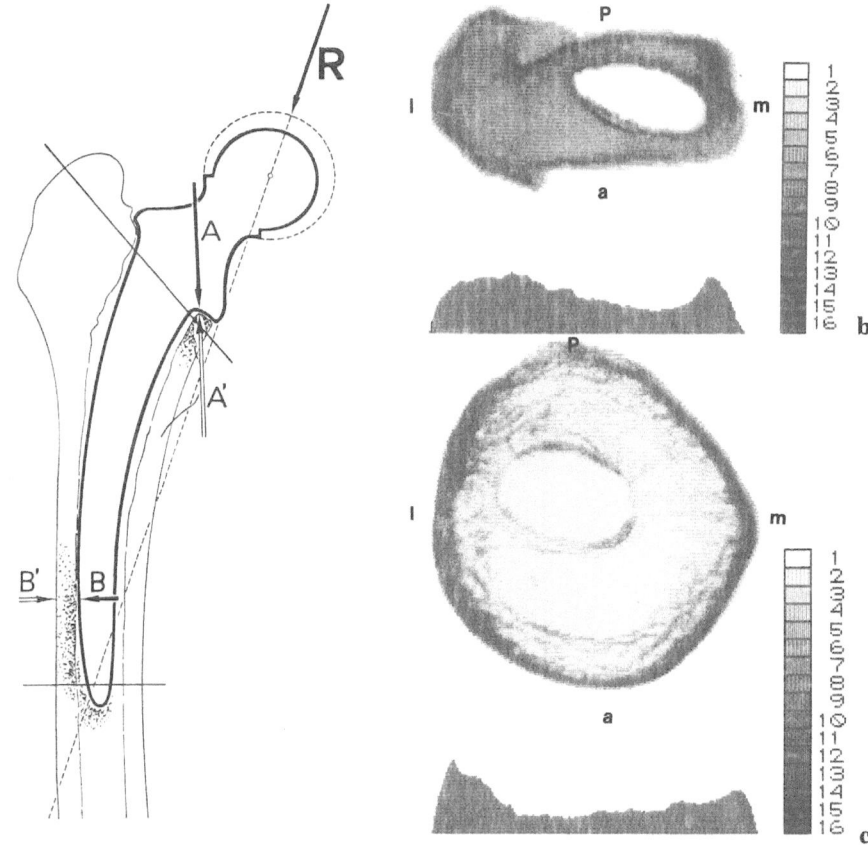

Fig. 8 a-c. Cementless implanted femoral endoprosthesis in an 84-year-old female. **a** Biomechanical analysis of the stress condition. *A*, pressure force at the proximal support (fulcrum); *B*, pressure of the stem against the lateral diaphyseal wall; *B'*, bone resistance against the force B; *R*, hip resultant. **b** Cross-sectional slice (5 mm thick) of the specimen, parallel to and immediately beneath the collar of the endoprosthesis. Niveau of the force-counter force reaction A, A' in **a**. Density distribution in the X-ray of **a**. Underneath the mass of bone material is summed up respective to a latero-medial baselines ("mass contraction"). The numbers *1-16* mark the zones of equal relative density. **c** Cross-sectional slice (5 mm thick) of the specimen, shown in **a**, taken at the level of the force — counter force reaction B, B'

rarefication would be considered to be caused by local overloading. If, on the other hand, the prothesis has been cemented firmly (in spite of the poor covering of the stem by the cement), then the proximal medial wall in the calcar area would be protected from stresses and the bone resorption may be explained by reaction to inactivity. The analysis of the bone section however, only confirms the loss of bone substance (Fig. 9b), and cannot aid to determine whether it is due to stress-protection or overloading.

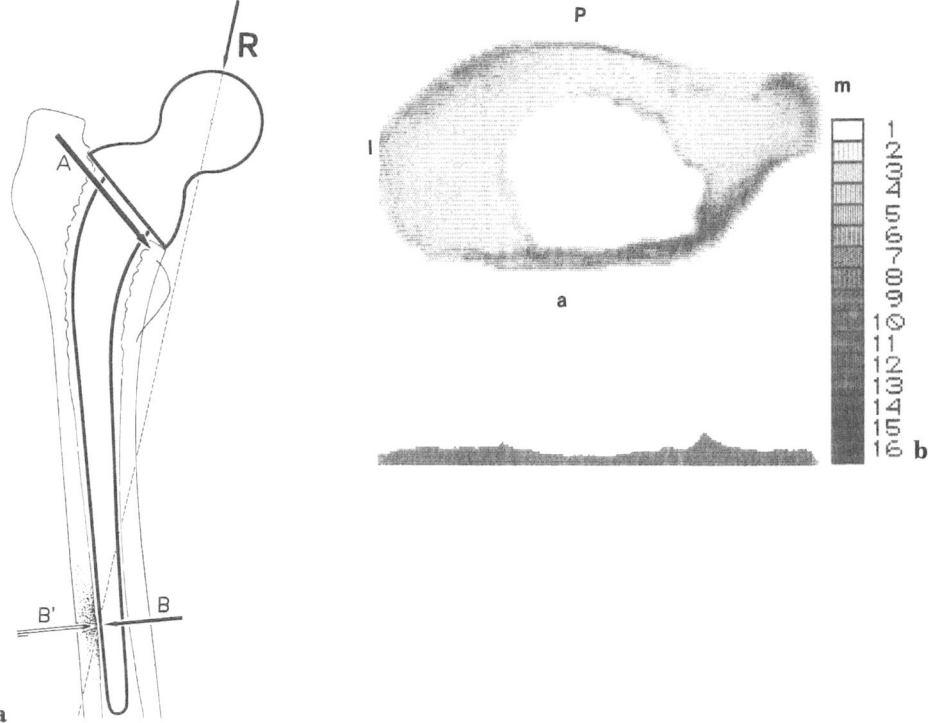

Fig. 9 a,b. Cemented femoral endoprosthesis in an 85-year-old female. **a** One possible biomechanical explanation of the stress situation. Same labels as in Fig. 8a. **b** Cross-sectional slice (5 mm thick) taken from the specimen just beneath and parallel to the collar of the prosthesis, showing the density distribution and mass contraction

Conclusions

Bone reacts on the implant of an endoprosthesis with remodelling in the sense of densification or rarefication of the bone material. These processes can be explained as the consequences of functional adaptation as described by Pauwels [2, 3]. In anatomical specimens, the effect of remodelling can be quantified.

References

1. Pauwels F (1973) Kurzer Überblick über die mechanische Beanspruchung des Knochens und ihre Bedeutung für die funktionelle Anpassung. Z Orthop 111: 681
2. Pauwels F (1976) Biomechanics of the normal and diseased hip. Springer, Berlin Heidelberg
3. Pauwels F (1980) Biomechanics of the locomotor apparatus. Springer, Berlin Heidelberg New York

4. Roux W (1895) Gesammelte Abhandlungen über Entwicklungsmechanik der Organismen, 1–2. Engelmann, Leipzig
5. Kummer B (1972) Biomechanics of bone: mechanical properties, functional structure, functional adaptation. In: Fung YC, Perrone N, Anliker M (eds) Biomechanics: its foundations and objectives. Prentice Hall, Englewood Cliffs, pp 237–271
6. Kummer B (1975) Biomechanical aspects of the total hip prosthesis. San Diego Biomedical symposium
7. Kummer B (1984) Die Beanspruchung des Femur durch implantierte Endoprothesen. In: Rahmanzahdeh, Faensen F (eds) Hüftgelenksendoprothetik, herausgeg. Springer, Berlin, pp 45–53
8. Kummer B (1985) Kraftfluß Prothese — Femur: Anpassugs- und Überlastungsreaktionen des Knochens. In: Maaz B, Menge M (eds) Aktueller Stand der zementfreien Hüftendoprothetik, Symposion, 1985, Düsseldorf. Thieme, Stuttgart
9. Kummer B (1986) Zur Beanspruchung der normalen Hüftgelenkspfanne und des Implantatlagers bei zementierter Gelenksendoprothese. 8th München Symposion experimenteile, Orthopädie. Thieme, Stuttgart

Management of Femoral Bone Stock Deficiency in Total Hip Replacement

Hugh P. Chandler[1]

Summary. Forty-three femoral grafts were used to reconstruct femoral deficiency in revision total hip replacement. Allografts were used in the majority of cases but were always supplemented by autograft. Grafts were used to reconstruct deficiencies of the calcar, cortical perforation, fractures about or below the stem of the femoral component and for massive proximal deficiency of the metaphysis and diaphysis of the femur. These reconstructions were major procedures and complications were significant but comparable to those described for other revision surgery. The infection rate was 5.4%

Introduction

In recent years we have seen an increasing number of patients with complex femoral deficiencies, usually associated with failed total hip replacements. In the past, many surgeons have advocated more massive femoral components used with cement, but reconstruction when these fail can be very difficult. Distally sintered components can cause significant stress shielding. We prefer to reconstruct these defects with bone grafts. Our experience now consists of 37 patients with 43 femoral grafts. There were 23 females and 14 males, with an average age of 60 years. Mean follow-up was 19 months (6–67 months). Sixteen patients had isolated femoral grafts and 27 patients had femoral and acetabular grafts. Most of the grafts were undertaken for revision surgery of failed cemented total hip replacements.

Allografts were used in the majority of cases and in only two instances were autografts used alone, but all allografts were supplemented with autogenous bone from the iliac crest, from the femoral head (if available), or from reamings from the acetabulum. Seven of the grafts were femoral heads obtained from previous total hip surgeries, while 34 were allografts harvested from cadavers under strict asepsis. All grafts were cultured prior to freezing at $-80°C$. The Harris hip rating system was used to evaluate cases before and after surgery. At surgery, every attempt was made to ensure stability of the reconstructions, and therefore, postoperative management was similar to that of primary total hip replacement. Patients were placed in balanced suspension with Buck's traction only to protect the soft tissues (5 days mean). The average hospitalization was 14 days. Postoperatively, crutches were used for 6

---

[1] Ambulatory Care Center, Massachusetts General Hospital, Boston, Massachusetts, USA

weeks; then patients were encouraged to use a cane. The average time on a cane was 9 weeks.

The following are the femoral classifications of the main anatomical deficiencies dealt with:
1. Calcar deficiency
    a) Intramedullary
    b) Total deficiency
2. Trochanteric deficiency
3. Cortical thinning
4. Cortical perforation
5. Femoral fractures about or below the stem of a removal component
    a) Fractures of the patient's femur
    b) Fatigue fracture of an allograft
6. Circumferential deficiency of the metaphysis and proximal diaphysis
    a) Loss of the trochanter and metaphysis with a thin shell of the diaphysis remaining
    b) Total loss of the proximal femur

In many cases, combinations of more than one form of deficiency were encountered. Some selected cases will illustrate the problems and their management.

Calcar Deficiency

In our series, there were 4 isolated calcar defects and an additional 7 hips with a combination of calcar and other femoral defects, making a total of 11 hips (26%) with calcar problems. There are two patterns of calcar deficiency. With calcar intramedullary deficiency, a thin shell of bone remains at the periphery, but there is a central deficiency. With total calcar deficiency, the calcar is entirely deficient.

Calcar Intramedullary Deficiency

In the past, these problems have been treated by larger prostheses and/or more cement [1, 2]. We feel that grafting the defect with a femoral head, placed within the patulous proximal femur, offers a better solution [3].

Case 1. This 64-year-old man presented with a loose femoral component, 11 years after his original total hip replacement. The femoral component had subsided into varus with erosion of the central portion of the proximal femur, leaving only a thin rim of the calcar (Fig. 1a). He weighed 270 pounds. An allograft femoral head was shaped as a cylinder and was driven into the defect. A new medullary canal was fashioned laterally within this graft, forcing the new cemented component into valgus (Fig. 1b). Five years and 1 month later, the graft has incorporated, and there is no evidence of loosening of the total hip replacement (Fig. 1c). The patient still weighs 270 pounds and rates 98 on the Harris scale.

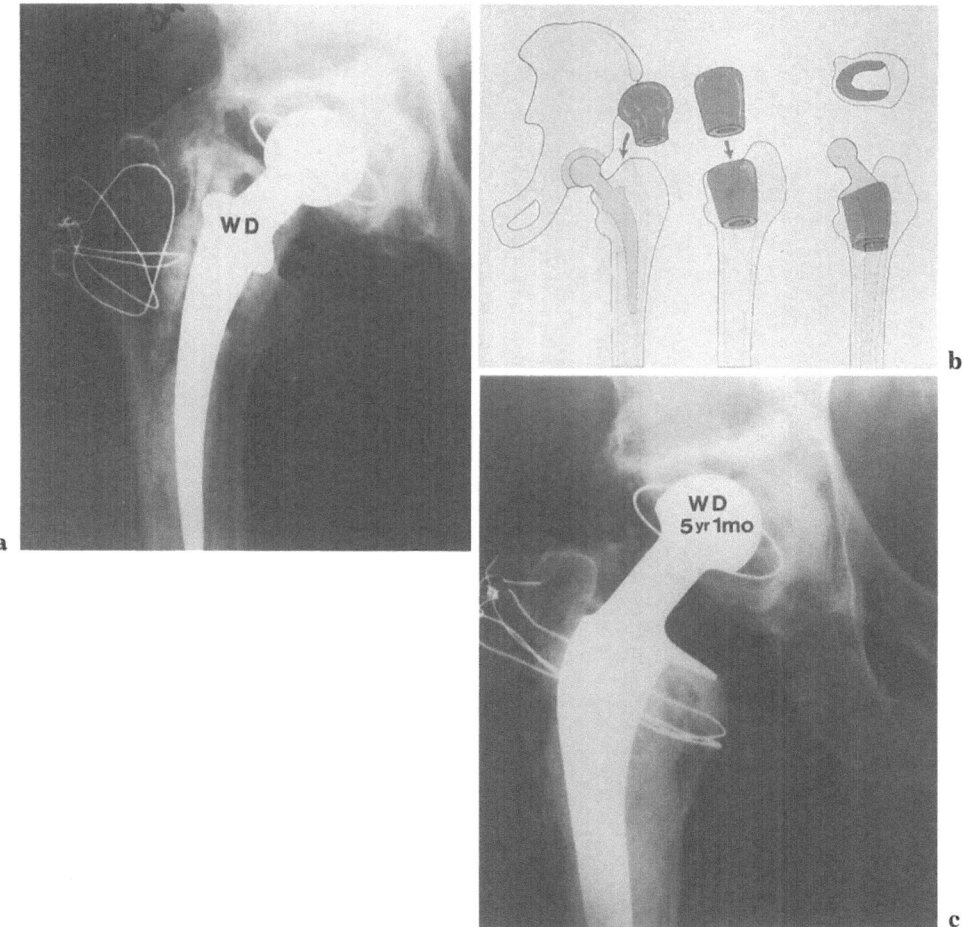

Fig. 1 a Preoperative view, **b** diagram, and **c** postoperative view of reconstruction surgery in case 1 (*WD*), a 64-year-old male

Total Calcar Deficiency

If the calcar is entirely absent, we prefer to use the calcar of an allograft femur, along with a distal strut which is used both for fixation (with circlage wires) and for reinforcement of cortical deficiency.

Case 2. This 69-year-old female had a failed femoral component which had subsided into varus. The tip had eroded the lateral femoral cortex (Fig. 2a, b). The acetabulum required grafting of a medial and superior intra-acetabular defect. An uncemented Harris-Galante cup was used. The absent femoral calcar was replaced by an allo-

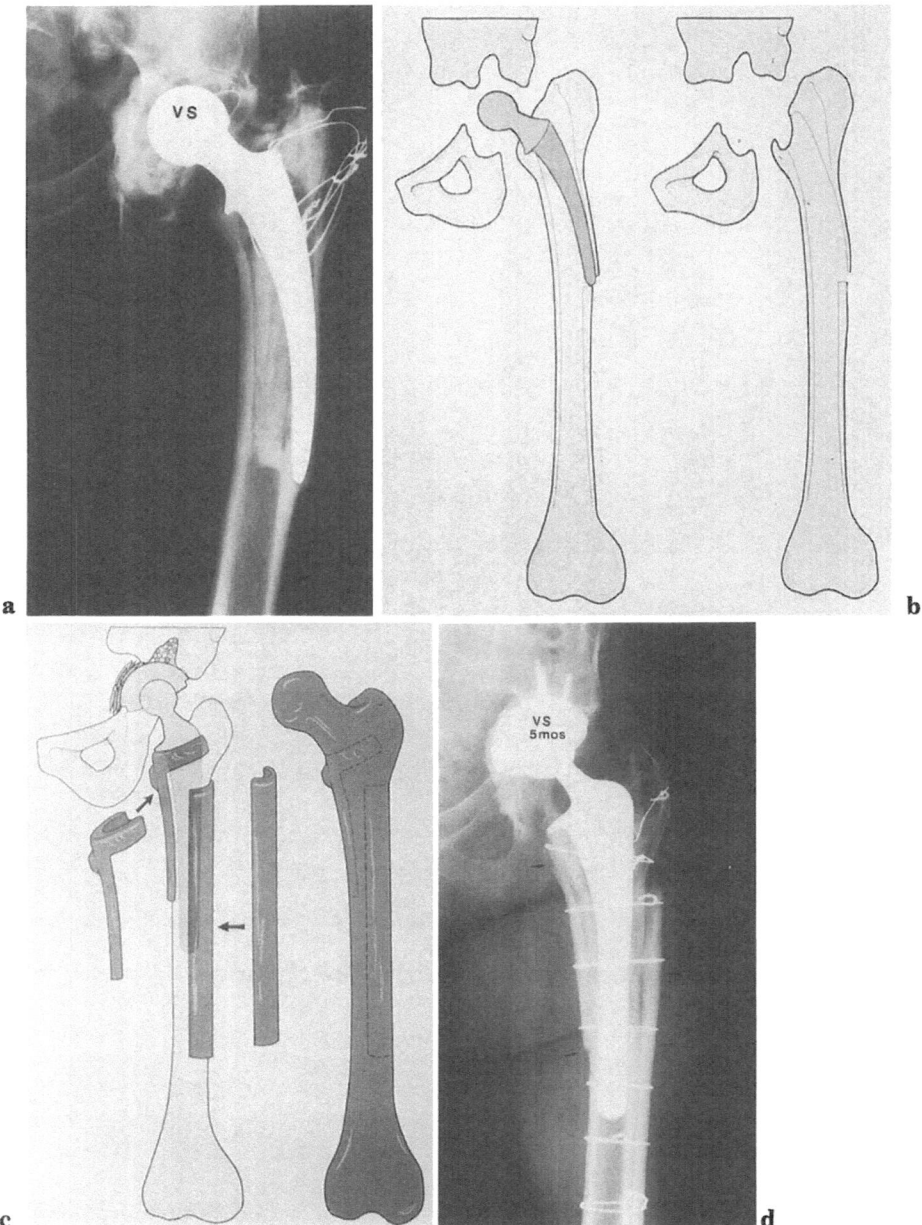

Fig. 2 a Preoperative view, **b, c** diagrams, and **d** postoperative view of reconstruction surgery in case 2(VS), a 69-year-old female

graft calcar in combination with a medial strut which reinforced the thin medial cortex and aided in fixation. The thin lateral cortex was reinforced by another allograft strut held with circlage wires. All grafts were supplemented by autogenous iliac crest strips (Fig. 2c). The patient was out of bed on day 3 and discharged at day 10, graduating to a cane at 6 weeks. She progressed to independent ambulation at 5 months, and radiographs at that time showed early incorporation (Fig. 2d). At 1 year and 4 months she reports no problems and rates 86.

Cortical Thinning and Cortical Perforation

In our series there were 7 hips with isolated perforation or thinning of the cortex and 14 that had these problems in combination with other defects, making a total of 21 hips (48%) with cortical deficiencies. In the past, many authors have recommended longer stems to bypass cortical defects [4]. Such implants can cause further cortical damage by stress shielding. We prefer to use massive cortical onlay grafts, held with circlage wires, to reinforce the deficient cortex. Standard length femoral components are satisfactory, and it is not necessary to bypass the defect with a longer term.

Case 3. This 53-year-old woman with Parkinson's disease had a resection arthroplasty in treatment for a staphylococcus epidermidis infection which occurred after a previous total hip replacement (Fig. 3a). The femoral shaft was perforated when the cement was removed (Fig. 3b). The lateral cortical defect was reconstructed by means of a femoral cortical allograft strut (Fig. 3c). A standard length uncemented Harris-Galante prosthesis was used (Fig. 3d). Because of the underlying Parkinson's disease, the hip dislocated and required closed reduction on 11 occasions. Despite the fact that the femoral stem did not bypass the defect, the femur did not fracture. The hip has not dislocated again since an anterior obturator neurectomy and an adductor tenotomy. At 3½ years the graft has joined with the cortex (Fig. 3e). The patient uses a walker because of her Parkinson's disease and rates only 74.

Standard length regular components were used in the majority of the 21 patients with cortical thinning or perforations, and there have not been any fractures through the areas of previously compromised cortex.

Femoral Fractures about or below a Femoral Component

In our series, there were 6 patients (14%) with fractures involving the femur in the presence of a total hip replacement stem. In the past, most authors have recommended traction treatment or replacing the femoral component with a longer stem [5, 6]. We prefer to reduce the fracture, fix it with circlage wires, and then reinforce the area with massive medial and lateral only femoral allograft struts which are held with circlage wires.

Case 4. This 70-year-old female was treated with a cemented long-stem component after a revision 4 years previously (Fig. 4a). Such components typically cause stress shielding. In her case, the femoral cortices were paper thin, and the well-cemented

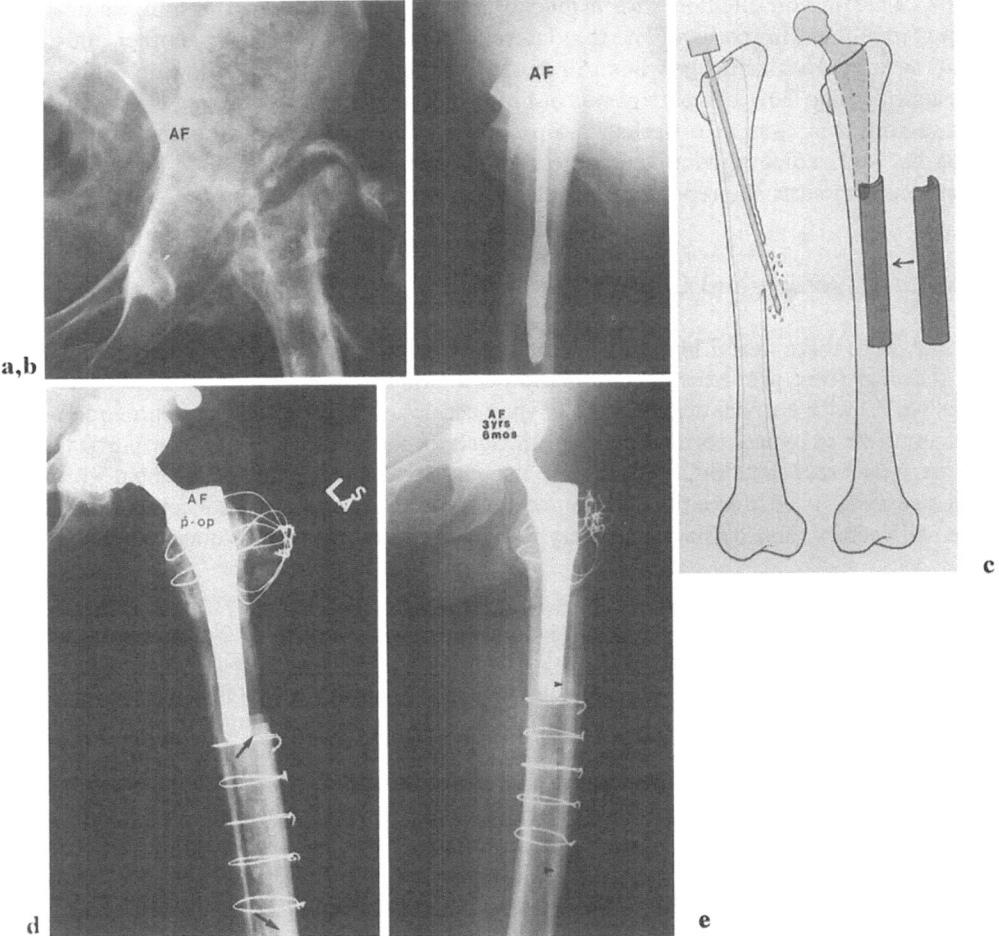

Fig. 3 a,b Preoperative views, **c** diagram, and **d, e** and postoperative views of reconstruction surgery in case 3(*AF*), a 53-year-old female

component could not have been removed without destroying the proximal femur. The patient was initially treated in traction, but because of concurrent medical problems, this was not well tolerated; and it was felt that the fracture should be surgically stabilized so that she could be mobilized. The fracture was fixed temporarily with two circlage wires (Fig. 4b), and then held with two massive femoral cortical allografts. The patient was able to get out of bed on day 2 and began partial weight bearing. The patient lived for 1 year, and then died of unrelated problems. Up to that time, she used a walker for balance only and was without pain. The fracture had united clinically and the graft appeared to be uniting radiographically at 8 months (Fig. 4c).

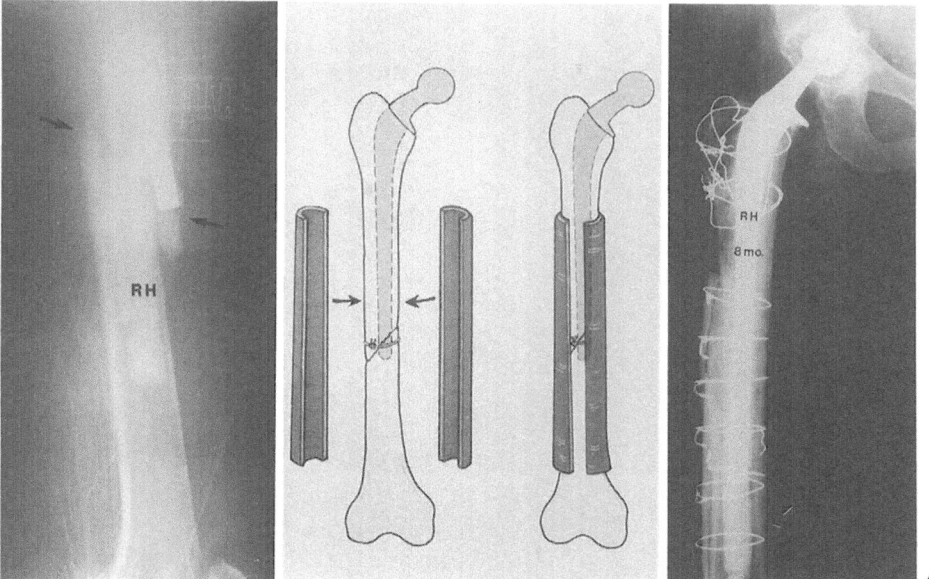

a,b   c

Fig. 4 a Preoperative view, **b** diagram, and **c** postoperative view of reconstruction surgery in case 4 (*RH*), a 70-year-old female

All at our patients that have been treated in this manner have united their fractures. The femoral component was replaced only if it was loose, and in these cases, standard length components were used.

Circumferential Deficiency of the Metaphysis and Diaphysis

In our series, there were 11 patients (26%) with massive proximal femoral loss. Other authors have recommended prostheses that replace the proximal femur or allografts used in conjunction with long-stemmed components [7–12]. We prefer to use a large proximal femoral allograft with a long distal strut used for fixation, as well as for reinforcement of deficient cortices. Stems should bypass the junction of the allograft and host bone by 8 cm. Standard length components are often satisfactory.

Case 5. This 62-year-old woman with a dysplastic hip had 4 previous unsuccessful mold arthroplasties. A custom long-stem Moore prosthesis was then inserted. The patient required two axillary crutches for the 22 years while this prosthesis was in place. At the time of reconstruction, there was major loss of acetabular bone stock, and there was dramatic stress shielding of her femur as well as a distal perforation (Fig. 5a, b). Because of the thin cortices, an intraoperative fracture of the femoral shaft occurred (Fig. 5c). The distal condyles of an allograft femur were used to reconstruct the dome of the acetabulum and the anterior and superior rim, and an-

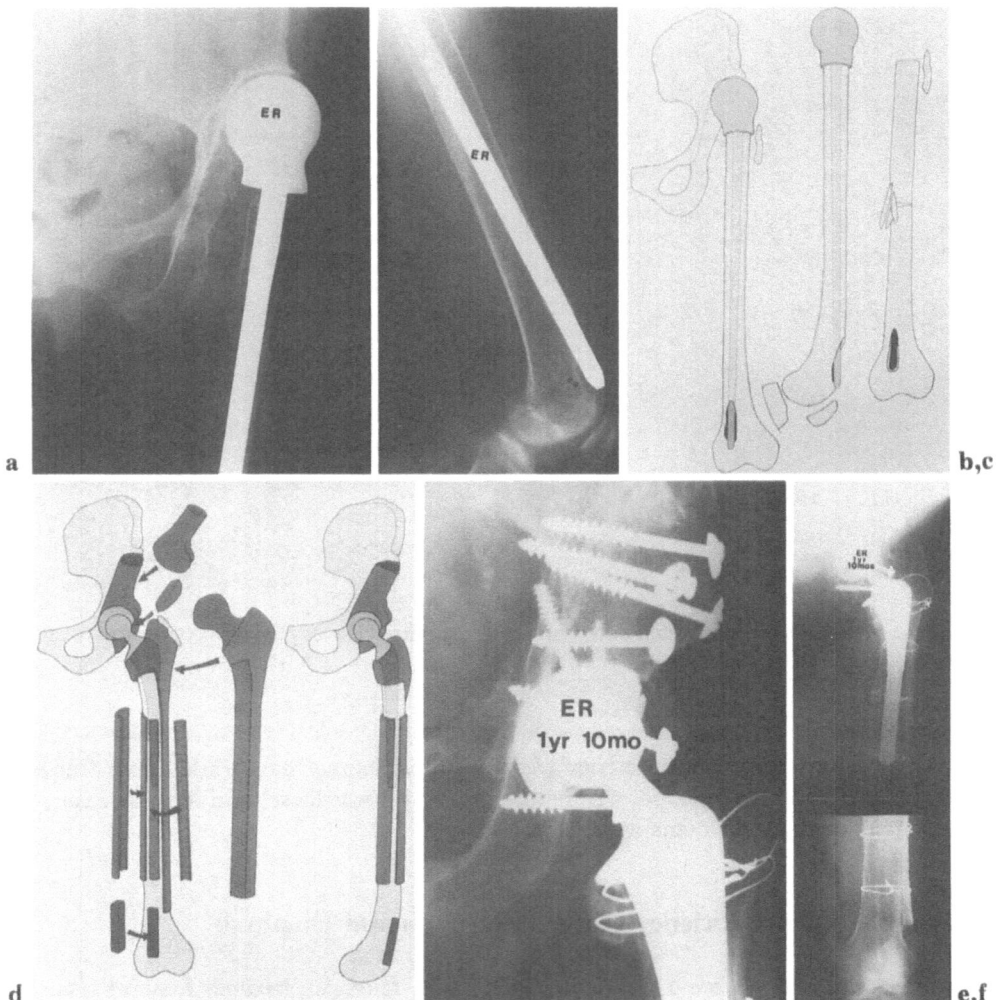

Fig. 5 a,b Preoperative views, **c, d** diagrams, and **e, f** postoperative views of reconstruction surgery in case 5 (*ER*), a 62-year-old female

other allograft was used to reconstruct the posterior acetabulum. The femur was reconstructed using a proximal allograft femur with a side strut which extended to the knee. The fracture was dealt with by two other allograft cortical struts. An uncemented standard-length femoral component was used (Fig. 5d). At 1 year and 10 months, both the acetabular and femoral reconstructions appear to be doing well (Fig. 5e, f). The fracture of the femur is clinically united. The patient requires a cane because of weak abductors but has good motion and no pain. She rates 88.

Table 1. Total hip replacement complications

Complication	No. of cases
Intraoperative	
Fractured femur	6
Perforation of remoral shaft	4
Excessive blood loss	1
Peroneal Palsy	1
Postoperative	
Dislocation	10
Infection	2 (5.4%)
Acute	1
Hematogenous	1
Heterotopic ossification	4
Trochanteric avulsion	3
Phlebitis	4

Results and Complications

The Harris hip rating was used to evaluate all these patients. The average preoperative Harris rating for the series was 44 and postoperatively was 88. However, it should be reemphasized that these reconstructions were major procedures and complications were significant (Table 1).

In summary, for intramedullary calcar deficiency we prefer to use an allograft femoral head shaped to fit the proximal femoral canal. For total deficiency of the calcar, a calcar and distal strut from an ipsilateral allograft femur can be used. Fractures below or about a femoral component can be fixed with circlage wires and reinforced by massive cortical onlay grafts held with circlage wires. It is not necessary to bypass the fracture with a long-stem component. Thinning or perforation of the femoral cortex can be treated with onlay cortical struts and standard-length components. Circumferential loss of the proximal metaphysis and diaphysis can be reconstructed using a large proximal femoral allograft with a long distal strut and with a stem that bypasses the junction of the allograft and host bone by 8 cm. We feel that the bone-grafting techniques described here offer the best solution to these difficult examples of bone stock deficiency in total hip replacement.

References

1. Turner RH, Emerson RH (1982) Femoral revision total hip arthroplasty. In: Turner RH, Scheller AO (eds) Revision total hip arthroplasty. Greene & Stratton, New York, p. 97
2. Harris WH, Allen JR (1981) The calcar replacement femoral component for total hip arthroplasty. Clin Orthop 157: 215–224
3. Chandler HP, Penenberg BL (1984) Autografts and allografts in total hip replacement. (science exhibit) Am Acad Orthop Surg
4. Scott RD, Turner RH (1975) Avoiding complications with long stem total hip replacement arthroplasty. J Bone Joint Surg 57: A722

5. Johansson JE, McBroom R, Barrington TW (1981) Fracture of the ipsilateral femur in patients with total hip replacement. J Bone Joint Surg 63: A1435–A1442
6. Scott RD, Schiltz JD (1982) Femoral fractures and revision arthroplasty. In: Turner RH, Scheller AO (eds) Revision total hip arthroplasty. Greene and Stratton, New York, p 127
7. Sim FH, Chao EYS (1981) Hip salvage by proximal femoral replacement. J Bone Joint Surg 63: A1228–A1239
8. Scheller AD, D'Errico J (1982) Hip biomechanics and prosthetic design and selection. In: Turner RH, Scheller AD (eds) Revision total hip arthroplasty. Greene and Stratton, New York, p 67
9. McGann W, Mankin HJ, Harris WH (1986) Massive allografting for severe failed total hip replacement. J Bone Joint Surg 68: A1–A12
10. Makley JT (1985) The use of allografts to reconstruct intercalcar defects of long bones. Clin Orthop 197: 58–75
11. Mnaymneh W, Malinin T, Head WC, Borja F, Berkhalter W, Reyes F, Zych G, Ballard A (1986) Massive osteoarticular allografts in non-tumorous conditions. (science exhibit) Am Acad Orthop Surg
12. Head WC, Malinin TI Berklacich F (1987) Freeze-dried proximal femur allografts in revision total hip arthroplasty. Clin Orthop 215: 109–120

Bone Grafting of Acetabular Deficiencies in Total Hip Replacement

ALAN H. WILDE and BERNARD N. STULBERG[1]

Summary. Bony deficiencies in the acetabulum are not infrequently encountered in total hip replacement. Deficiencies occur as the result of disease, trauma or previous surgery. Bone deficiency as the result of disease can be seen in rheumatoid arthritis, idiopathic protrusio acetabuli, congenital dislocation of the hip or acetabular dysplasia, cerebral palsy, coxa vara, arthrogryposis, or Ollier's disease. Fracture dislocation of the hip can produce severe distortion of the pelvis requiring major reconstruction of the acetabulum. Some of the largest deficiencies can be seen following failed cemented total hip arthroplasties. Protrusio acetabuli can occur following hemi-arthroplasty of the hip.

Methods of Compensating for Acetabular Bone Loss

The available methods of correcting bone loss in the acetabulum are:
1. Methyl methacrylate bone cement
2. Prosthetic replacement
3. Bone grafting.

Cement has been used to fill in bone defects in the acetabulum in the past. As cement lacks the same mechanical properties as bone, there is a risk of failure due to inadequate support of the prosthesis. Figure 1 shows an intrapelvic protrusion of the femoral head. A total hip replacement was performed (Fig. 2) using radiolucent cement to fill in the acetabular defect. Within 3 years the floor of the acetabulum had given way and the cup and cement migrated into the true pelvis (Fig. 3). Various prostheses have been made to repair defects in the acetabulum and protrusio rings and deeper protrusio cups are available. However, these devices can also fail when used alone without adequate bone support.

Bone grafting has the advantage of correcting the problem using a biologic material which can provide the support needed. The bone grafts that can be used are autogenous from the patient or an allograft. Autogenous bone has many advantages. Cancellous autogenous bone grafts heal rapidly and are almost completely replaced by host bone. They also do not undergo resorption due to an allergic response. Allografts heal to host bone although union to the host bone typically requires 1 year. Fresh-frozen allograft bone is not completely replaced by host bone but does retain its mechanical strength for prolonged periods. Freeze-dried bone has the advantage

---

[1] Department of Orthopedic Surgery, The Cleveland Clinic Foundation, Cleveland, Ohio, USA

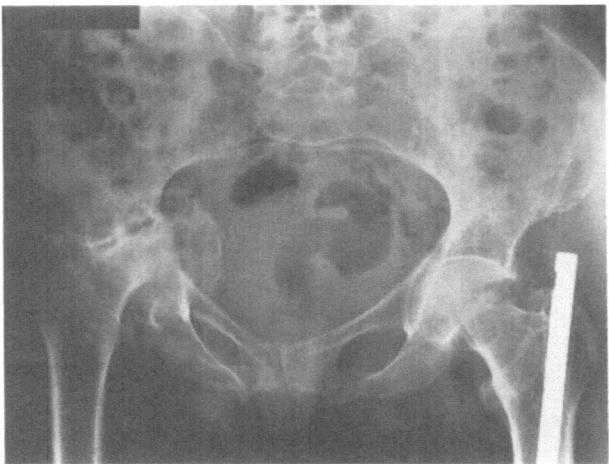

Fig. 1. Acetabular protrusion of the femoral head into the true pelvis

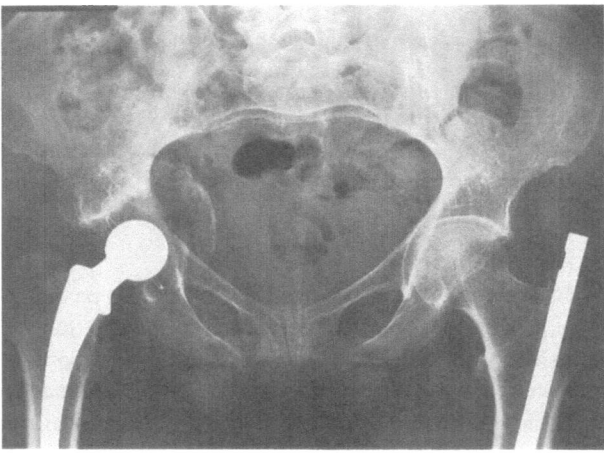

Fig. 2. Anteroposterior roentgenograms of both hips of the patient in Fig 1. A total hip replacement using radiolucent cement. Additional cement was used in the floor of the acetabulum to fill the acetabular defect

of lessened antigenicity but lacks the strength of fresh-frozen allografts. In the repair of major acetabular defects, solid grafts are required for support. The use of morsel-ized cancellous bone to replace a major defect in the superior weight-bearing dome of the acetabulum is likely to result in collapse of the graft.

In primary total hip replacements, the patient's femoral head can be utilized as a source of bone for the acetabular defect. In protrusio acetabuli, traumatic arthritis from a fracture dislocation, congenital dislocation of the hip, cerebral palsy, coxa

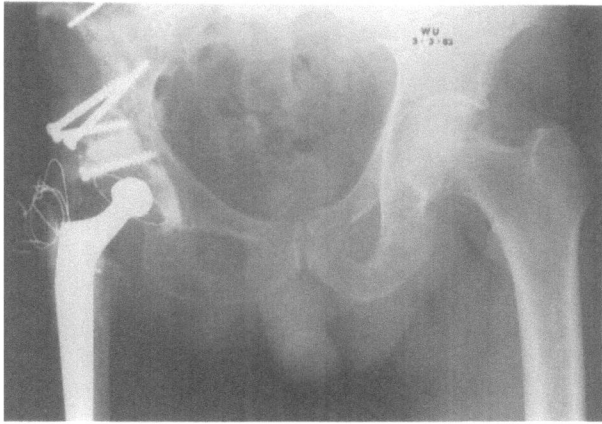

Fig. 3. The acetabular component of the patient in Figs. 1 and 2 has migrated into the true pelvis

vara and arthrogryposis, the patient's femoral head usually suffices to repair the bone loss in the acetabulum.

A problem arises when there has been a previous hip reconstruction and there is no source of bone from the patient large enough to fill the defect. In this situation, an allograft can be used. We prefer to use fresh-frozen allografts which have been retrieved from cadavers. The bone is stored at $-70°C$. It is cultured at the time of harvest and again at the time of use. If the cultures are positive, the bone is discarded. Blood can be taken from the deceased to test for acquired immune deficiency syndrome. Fresh-frozen bone also has greater strength than freeze-dried bone. We have used cadaver femoral heads, half of a distal femoral condyle, the distal tibia or talus to reconstruct acetabular defects in cases of failed total hip replacement.

Preparation of the Allograft

The allograft is warmed to room temperature in sterile saline or Ringer's lactate solution. All soft tissue, articular cartilage and subchondral plate are removed. The allograft is shaped with a saw or rongeur to fill the defect in the acetabulum. At times the allograft can be wedged in tightly so that internal fixation is unnecessary. Usually however it is necessary to use partially threaded 6.5 mm AO cancellous acetabular screws. The screws are inserted at the periphery of the graft into the ilium. Two or 3 screws are countersunk so they will not impinge on an acetabular reamer. A flexible drill is invaluable for the placement of the screws.

The graft and acetabulum are reamed for an appropriate size cup. Any defects between the allograft and the acetabulum are filled with additional cancellous bone. Bone cement can then be inserted, pressurized and a cup inserted at the proper

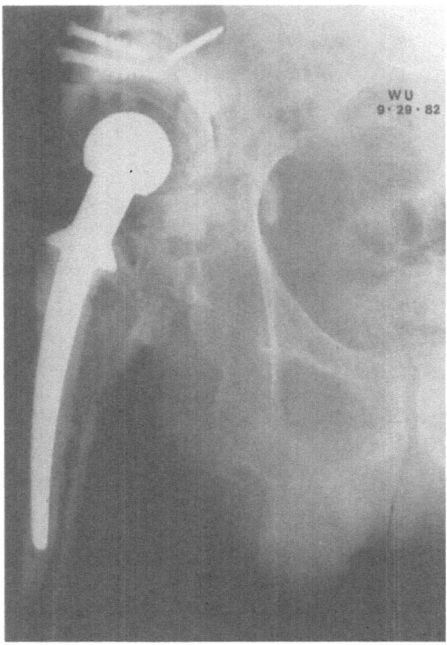

WU
9·29·82

Fig. 4 Anteroposterior roentgenogram of a patient after cemented total hip replacement. The acetabular component in the false acetabulum has loosened

angle. Fig. 4 shows a failed total hip replacement in a patient with congenital dislocation of the hip. The cup, which had been placed in the false acetabulum, has loosened. Fig. 5 shows the reconstruction using an allograft which has been internally fixed with AO screws. The cup has been placed in the true acetabulum.

If the acetabular component of a cemented total hip replacement migrates through the medial wall of the acetabulum into the true pelvis, as in Fig. 3, the possibility exists of injury to the pelvic vessels, bowel or bladder (Fig. 6). It is recommended that an arteriogram of the pelvic vessels, intravenous pyelogram, and barium enema are performed.

Results of Bone Grafting Acetabular Deficiencies

Revisions of Total Hip Replacement

We have reported the results of 21 hip replacements using fresh-frozen femoral head allografts in failed cemented total hip replacements. The shortest follow-up was 2 years and the longest was 4 year, with an average follow-up of 3.5 years. The grafts were evaluated using roentgenograms and scintigraphic studies. The scintigraphic studies included planar scans and single photon emission computed tomography (SPECT). The SPECT scanner makes 64 images of the hip joint in a 360° arc. This procedure is ideal for the evaluation of the allograft-host bone interface. In 20 of the 21 cases, the allograft had united with the host bone. There was only one collapse of the allograft, an incidence of 5.8%. There were no infections in this series.

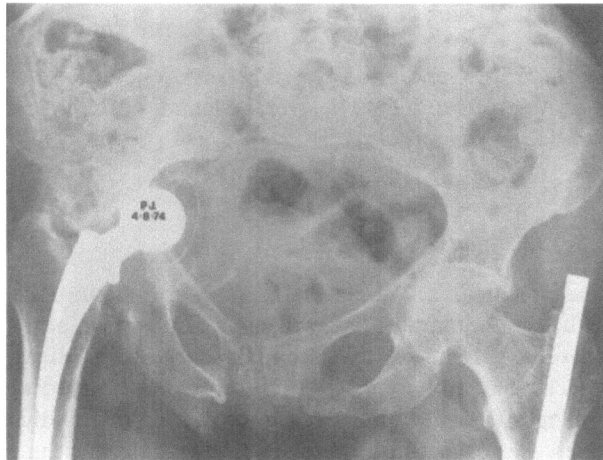

Fig. 5. Anteroposterior roentgenogram of both hips shows the hip reconstruction of the patient in Fig. 4, using an acetabular allograft internally fixed with AO screws. The acetabular component has been placed in the true acetabulum

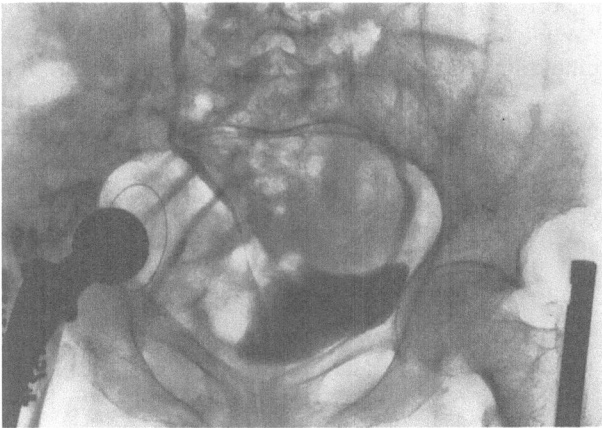

Fig. 6. Anteroposterior roentgenogram showing the migration of the acetabular component throught the medial wall of the acetabulum into the true pelvis

Protrusio Acetabuli

McCollum et al [1] reported the results in 32 patients followed up for 2–8 years, using homologous and autogenous bone grafts. All grafts appeared to unite within 3 months. There were no infections. They stated that bone grafting was effective in arresting the progression of acetabular protrusion.

Congenital Dislocation of the Hip

In a report by Gerber and Harris [2] of 47 operations using the patient's own femoral head, all grafts united. The average length of follow-up was 7.1 years and the minimum follow-up was 5 years.

Discussion

Bone grafting in acetabular deficiencies in patients undergoing total hip replacement has been successful in primary cases of protrusio acetabuli, congenital hip dislocation or dysplasia and in secondary surgeries such as revision of failed total hip replacement. The majority of the grafts have healed whether they were autogenous or allografts. Autogenous grafts healed more rapidly than allografts and may be healed as soon as three months, whereas allografts may take as long as 12 months to unite. Autografts were more likely to be completely replaced by host bone. In allografts, necrotic bone can persist for prolonged periods and it is doubtful that the allografts are ever completely replaced. If allografts are to be used, proper methods of collection, storage and processing must be utilized. It is important also when using allografts to correct large acetabular defects, to use a solid allograft for support.

While reported results have been with the use of cemented cups, we have been accumulating experience using allografts and cementless cups. Fixation of the allograft to host bone as well as the cup to acetabulum are important if success is to be achieved with a cementless cup.

References

1. McColum DE, Nunley JA, Narrelson JM (1980) Bone grafting in total hip replacement for acetabular protrusion. J Bone Joint Surg 62A: 1065–1072
2. Gerber SD, Harris WH (1986) Femoral head autografting to augment acetabular deficiency in patients requiring total hip replacement. J Bone Joint Surg 68A: 1241–1248

Follow-up Results of Chiari Pelvic Osteotomy for Patients with Acetabular Dysplasia

KAZUSHI HIROHATA, RYOICHI SHIBA, and TOMIO SHIMIZU[1]

Summary. We performed the Chiari pelvic osteotomy on 230 hips with acetabular dysplasia between 1970 and 1986 at Kobe University Hospital. A supplementary procedure was also occasionally performed. Excluding the combined surgery cases, 131 hips were examined 3 to 16 years later (average follow-up: 7.1 years). Follow-up results were assessed using the hip score of the Japanese Orthopaedic Association. The best results were obtained in cases of prearthrosis and early osteoarthrosis in patients under 50 years. This osteotomy was an effective procedure for severe acetabular dysplasia with respect of relief of pain, improvement of gait, and ADL. The decision to perform this osteotomy is dependent upon the biomechanical evaluation of effectiveness, as there are both advantages and disadvantages.

Introduction

Chiari [1] first reported in 1955 a pelvic osteotomy procedure which was appropriate for unilateral congenital acetabular dysplasia of the hip in children aged 4–9 years, excluding those with narrowing of the hip joint space and severe deformity of the femoral head. However, over the last 30 years, this osteotomy has gained usage in the treatment of prearthrosis and osteoarthrosis secondary to congenital dislocation of the hip (CDH). Chiari himself [2] disregarded his original upper age limit and recently performing this osteotomy on a 69-year-old woman. We, too, have used it on patients with acetabular dysplasia of the hip as a single or a combined procedure [3]. This paper presents our indications, techniques, and results.

Indications

Age and Sex. Patients over the age of 50 with severe osteoporosis and soft tissue stiffness should be negated. There is no lower age limit, however, bilateral osteotomy is usually avoided in young nulliparous women to facilitate spontaneous delivery.

Preoperative mobility and stability in the involved hip. We require at least 70° of flexion and 10° of abduction. The hip must be sufficiently stable to maintain a standing position on the involved leg.

---

[1] Department of Orthopedic Surgery, Kobe University School of Medicine, Kobe, Japan

Radiographic assessment of acetabular dysplasia. There are three methods: use of a Sharp's angle of greater than 55°, a center-edge angle (CE angle) of less than 10°, and a faux profile angle (Lequesne) of less than 0°. The first two are taken, anterior-posterior (A-P) and the third laterally.

This procedure is also indicated for malformed acetabula with significant deformity of the femoral head secondary to Legg-Calvé-Perthes disease or neglected adult CDH; in these cases, it enlarges the contact area between the acetabulum and the femoral head. This procedure can be combined at the same time with the following procedures:

1. Transfer of the greater trochanter for coxa vara deformity
2. Intertrochanteric varus osteotomy for coxa valga
3. Cup and replacement arthroplasty for severe osteoarthritis of the hip
4. Arthrodesis for an infected hip.

Operative Procedures

Our technique employs a few modifications of the original Chiari procedure. Using an anterior approach, the tensor fascia latae, the gluteal muscles outside the iliac crest, and the abdominal and psoas muscles inside the iliac crest are partially detached. The greater sciatic notch is periosteally exposed. Special retractors were made for the characteristic structure of Japanese iliac bones, to prevent neurovascular damage while cutting through to the cortex of this bone. A well-trained assistant then inserts 2 retractors from the lateral and medial sides, and carefully keeps them overlapping during the procedure (Fig. 1). Using an air saw, the osteotomy is begun through the anterior iliac bone. After the osteotomy is complete, the distal

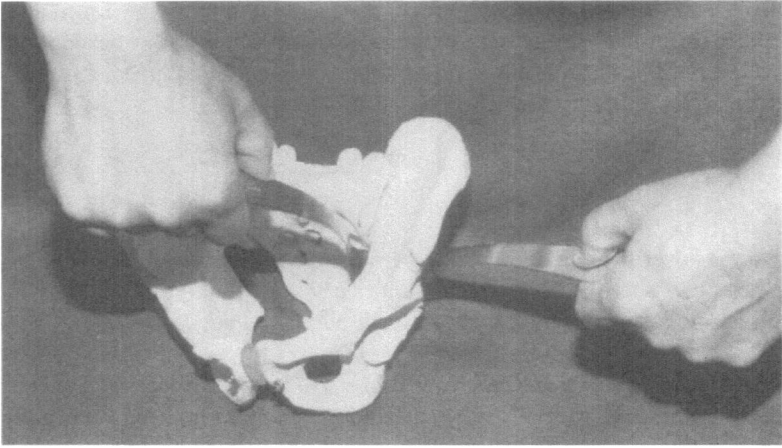

Fig. 1. Special retractors approach in the modified Chiari procedure to prevent neurovascular damage while cutting through the cortex

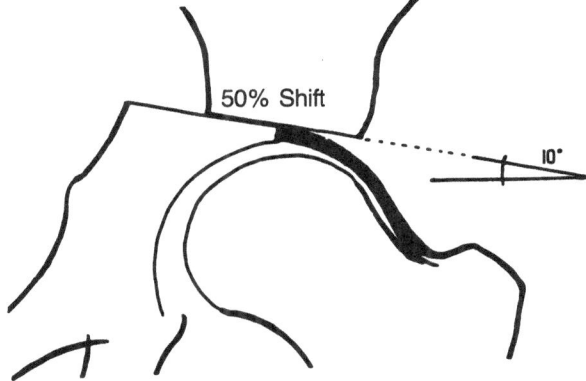

Fig. 2. Illustration showing the relationship of the new outer acetabular edge and the primitive edge, the osteotomy angle, and the level and degree of medial displacement (by Colton)

Table 1. Chiari pelvic osteotomy performed between 1970 and 1986 at Kobe University Hospital

Operation	No. of hips
Alone	177
With cup arthroplasty	41
With total hip replacement	8
With fusion	4
Total	230 hips (220 Cases)*

*Female (191 cases, 198 hips); Male (29 cases, 32 hips)

fragment is displaced medially and both fragments are transfixed with two kirschner-wires. The wound is then closed. Casting is unnecessary. Fig. 2 shows the relationship between the new outer acetabular edge and the primitive edge, as well as the osteotomy angle and the level and degree of medial displacement. In the ideal Chiari osteotomy, just above the capsular attachment, an angle of 10° is cut upwards and inwards, and displaced by a distance of 50% the width of the ilium (as suggested by Colton [4]).

We performed Chiari pelvic osteotomies on 191 women and 29 men with acetabular dysplasia between 1970 and 1986 at Kobe University Hospital (Table 1). Of these, 177 patients underwent the osteotomy alone and 53 underwent another procedure in combination. The average age was 33.8 years (range, 7–52). The average follow-up period was 7.0 years (range, 3–16). We were able to assess 131 (109 female, 22 male) cases using the scoring criteria of the Japanese Orthopaedic Association (the JOA hip score). Table 2 shows the JOA hip scores before osteotomy and the total number of patients in each age range. The JOA hip score was used to evaluate pain (Fig. 3),

Table 2. Patient profile and JOA hip score in 131 hips

Age (years)	Hip	JOA score
7– 9	13	95.3 ± 5.1
10–19	30	84.0 ± 12.2
20–29	25	80.0 ± 9.6
30–39	32	77.5 ± 7.0
40 and over	31	65.6 ± 16.6

JOA, Japan Orthopedics Association

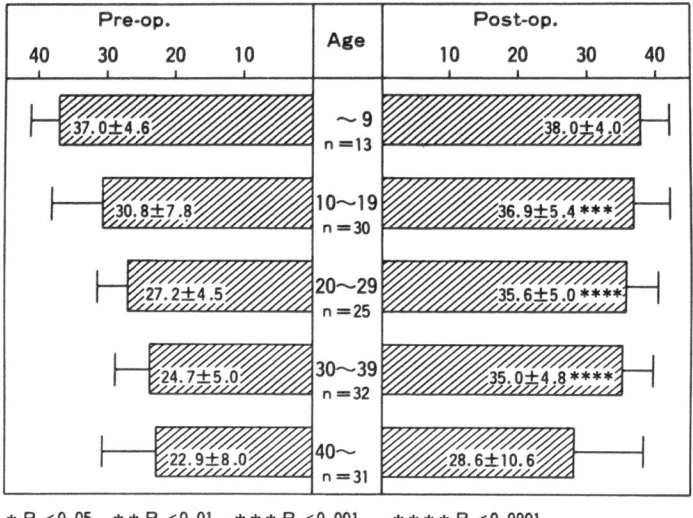

$*$ P <0.05 $**$ P <0.01 $***$ P <0.001 $****$ P <0.0001

Fig. 3. Pain score as assessed by the JOA criteria before (*Pre-op.*) and after (*Post-op.*) osteotomy in 131 patients

range of motion (Fig. 4), walking ability and gait (Fig. 5), and activities of daily living (ADL) (Fig. 6). Figure 7 summarizes the results. Figure 8 shows the radiographic procedure for the following assessments:

1. Comparison of the two lever arms of the abductor system before and after surgery
2. Sharp's angle, CE angle, and faux profile angle
3. Degree of medial displacement
4. Osteotomy level.

These results are shown in Figs. 9–12 and Table 3.

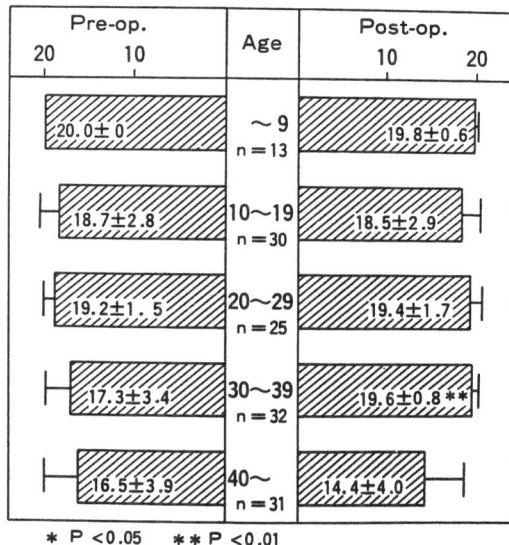

Fig. 4. Range of motion as assessed by the JOA criteria before (*Pre-op.*) and after (*Post-op.*) osteotomy in 131 patients

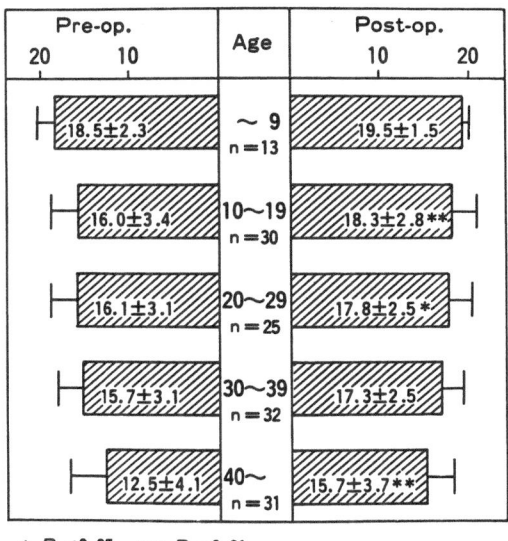

Fig. 5. Walking ability and gait as assessed by the JOA criteria before (*Pre-op.*) and after (*Post-op*) osteotomy in 131 patients

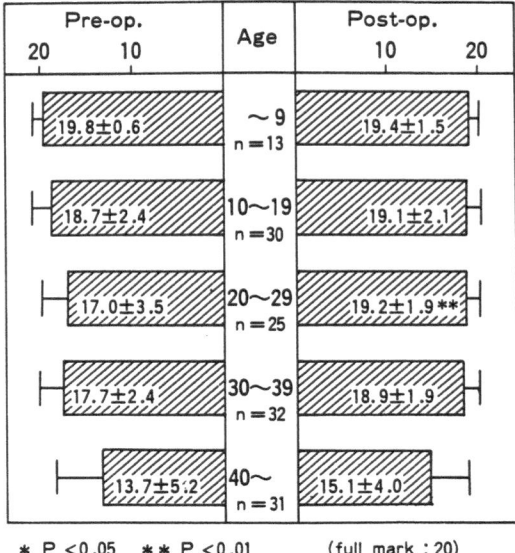

* P <0.05   ** P <0.01   (full mark : 20)

Fig. 6. Activities of daily living as assessed by the JOA criteria before (*Pre-op.*) and after (*Post-op.*) osteotomy in 131 patients

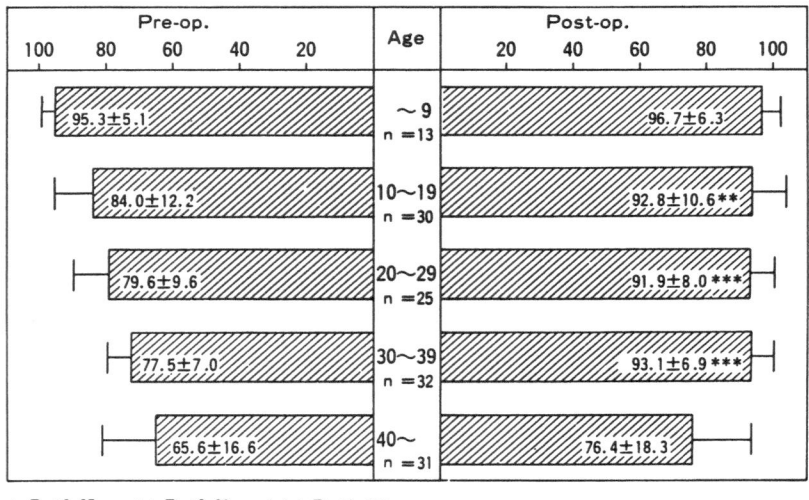

* P <0.05   ** P <0.01   *** P <0.001

Fig. 7. Summary of the *Pre-op.* and *Post-op.* Results of the assessments based on the JOA criteria of Chiari pelvic osteotomy in 131 dysplastic hips

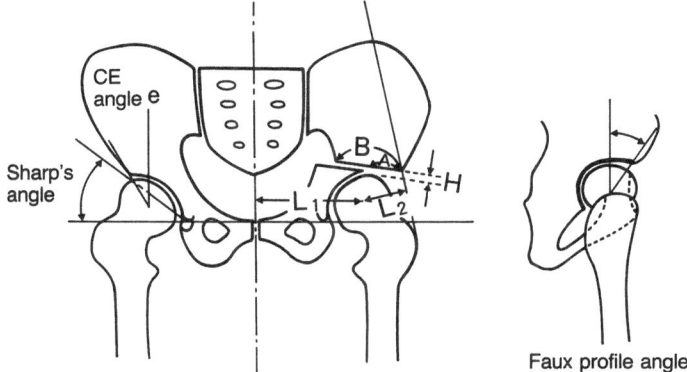

Fig. 8. Radiographic assessment procedure of determining *Sharp's angle*, *CE angle*, and *faux profile angle*. L_1/L_2, Ratio of lever arm length; $A/B \times 100$, percentage of displacement; H, osteotomy level above the head

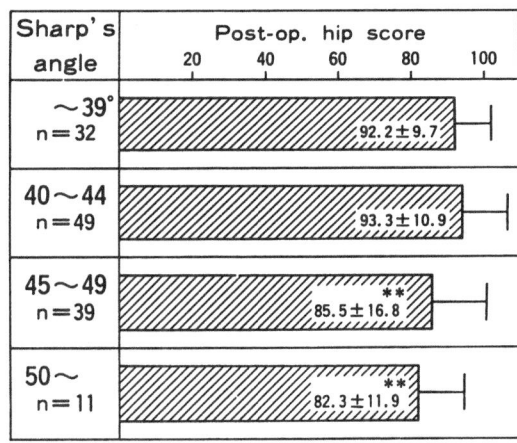

Fig. 9. Sharp's angle and total post-operative JOA hip score after osteotomy

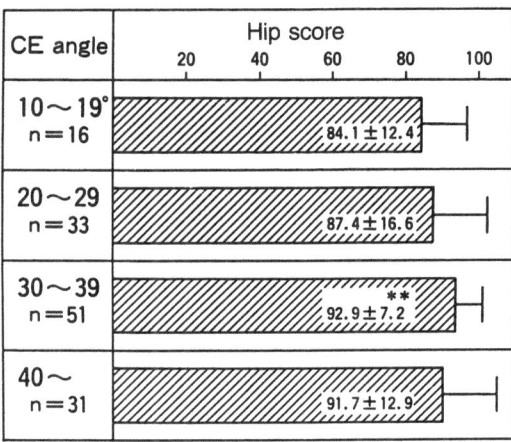

Fig. 10. CE angle and total post-operative JOA hip score after osteotomy

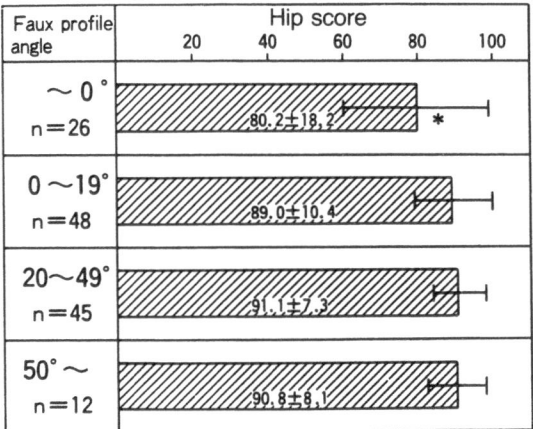

Fig. 11. Faux profile angle at follow-up and total post-operative JOA hip score after osteotomy

* P <0.01

** at follow-up

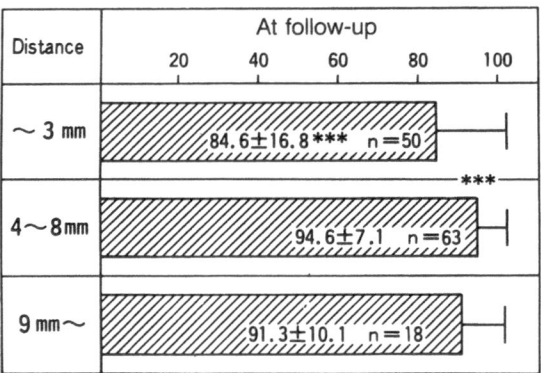

Fig. 12 Distance from the osteotomy line to femoral head and hip sore at follow-up

*** P <0.001

Table 3. Relationship of postoperative results and the ratio of the medial to the lateral arm of lever

Ratio		Total hip scores
%	No. of hips	
30–39	5	84.2 ± 11.7
40–49	23	84.8 ± 16.0
50–59	32	90.8 ± 11.7
60–69	15	93.9 ± 7.8*
≥ 70	8	98.8 ± 3.3**

* P<0.05
** P<0.01

Case Reports

Case 1. A young adult male with congenital acetabular dysplasia of the left hip (Fig. 13). The patient underwent the Chiari pelvic osteotomy at age of 15 due to fatigue pain around the hip. Thirteen years later, he was free from pain and had an excellent hip score.

Case 2. Early osteoarthrosis of the hip secondary to CDH (Fig. 14). This 47-year-old woman underwent the Chiari pelvic osteotomy of the left hip. Before osteotomy her complaints were severe hip pain, moderate limitation of hip motion, severe gait disturbance, and ADL problems. Her total hip score was 32 points below normal before surgery. After surgery this score increased gradually by 87 points over the subsequent 11 years. Radiography revealed that the cyst and bony sclerosis had disappeared and the joint space reappeared.

Case 3. Severe osteoarthrosis of the hip secondary to CDH (Fig. 15). Before surgery, the patient, a 43-year-old female, had to walk with a limp and severe pain. Her preoperative hip score was 59. She underwent the Chiari procedure combined with Cup arthroplasty. Six years later, she had no pain, could walk more than 30 min with only a slight limp, and had a hip score of 87.

Case 4. A supplementary Chiari pelvic osteotomy for late osteoarthrosis of the right hip secondary to CDH in the aged (Fig. 16). Before surgery, the ADL of this 56-year-old female was sharply reduced by severe hip pain and she had a total hip score of 55 points. She underwent the Chiari procedure combined with bipolar femoral head replacement. Two years later her pain was completely gone and she returned to work without any disturbance in walking ability or ADL, and a hip score of 95. Radiography revealed that the joint space reappeared and the subchondral sclerosis disappeared.

Discussion

Despite past age restrictions, the Chiari procedure can now be performed on adults as well as children. It is still best, however, for patients with acetabular dysplasia who are younger than 50. Since most elderly patients have stiff joints and ligaments in the pelvic ring, it is difficult to move the distal fragments much enough medially. Further, their osteoporosis delays bone healing, which is a contraindication of this osteotomy.

Women have CDH more often than men. Kotz et al. [5, 6] reported the manner in which this complicates child-birth. They studied nulliparous women who had undergone this procedure and found that 37 had delivered 53 babies, of which 83% had been spontaneously delivered and 17% required a Kaiser incision. The nulliparous women under our care have requested not to be subject to bilateral Chiari pelvic osteotomy, but some have undergone unilateral procedures after consulation with a gynecologist.

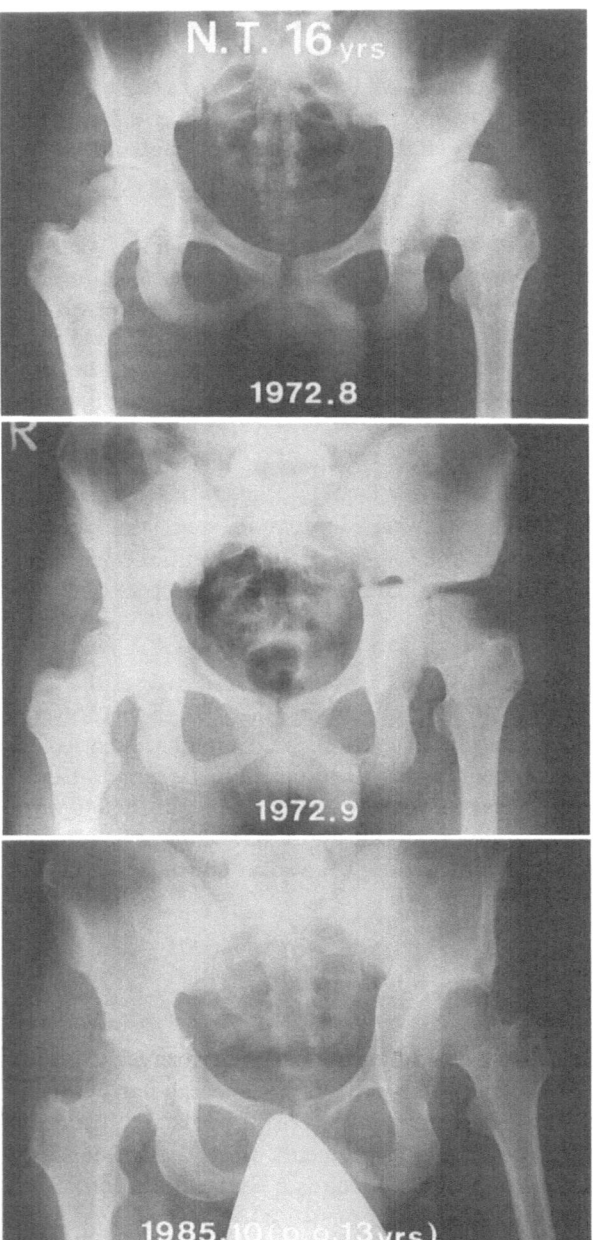

Fig. 13. Radiographic pictures of a 15-year-old male with congenital acetabular dysplasia of the left hip (*top*). At the 13-year follow-up (*bottom*) he was free from pain

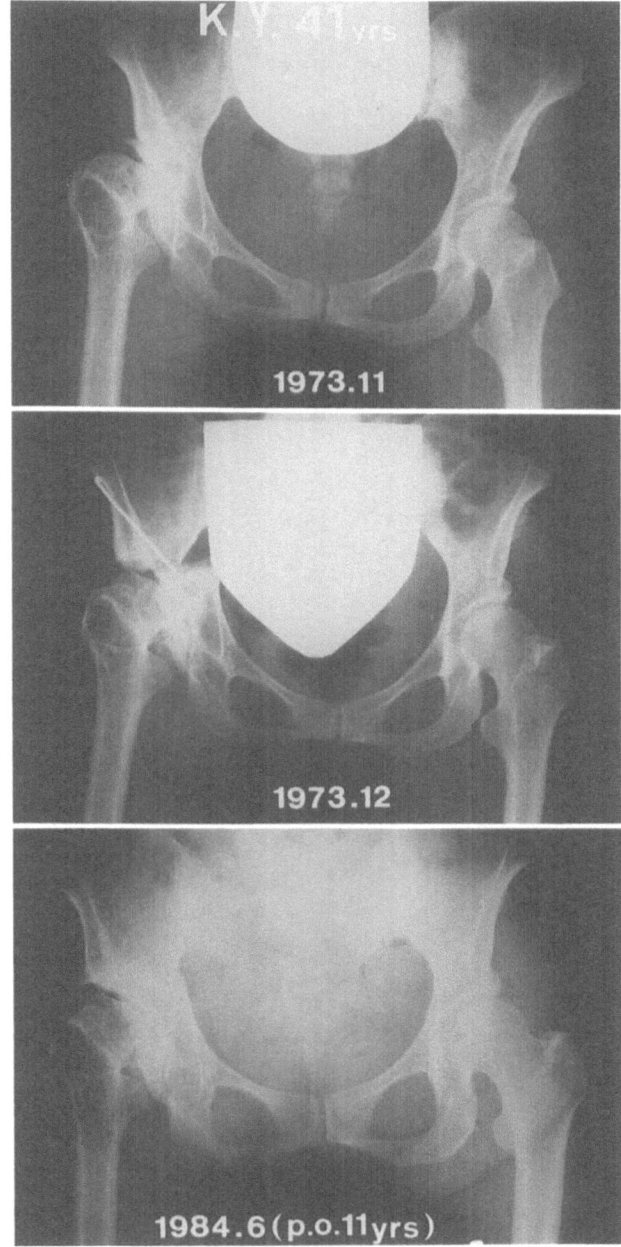

Fig. 14. Early osteoarthrosis of the left hip (*top*) in a 47-year-old female who underwent the Chiari pelvic osteotomy (*middle*). At the 11-year follow-up (*bottom*), the cyst and bony sclerosis had disappeared and the joint space reappeared

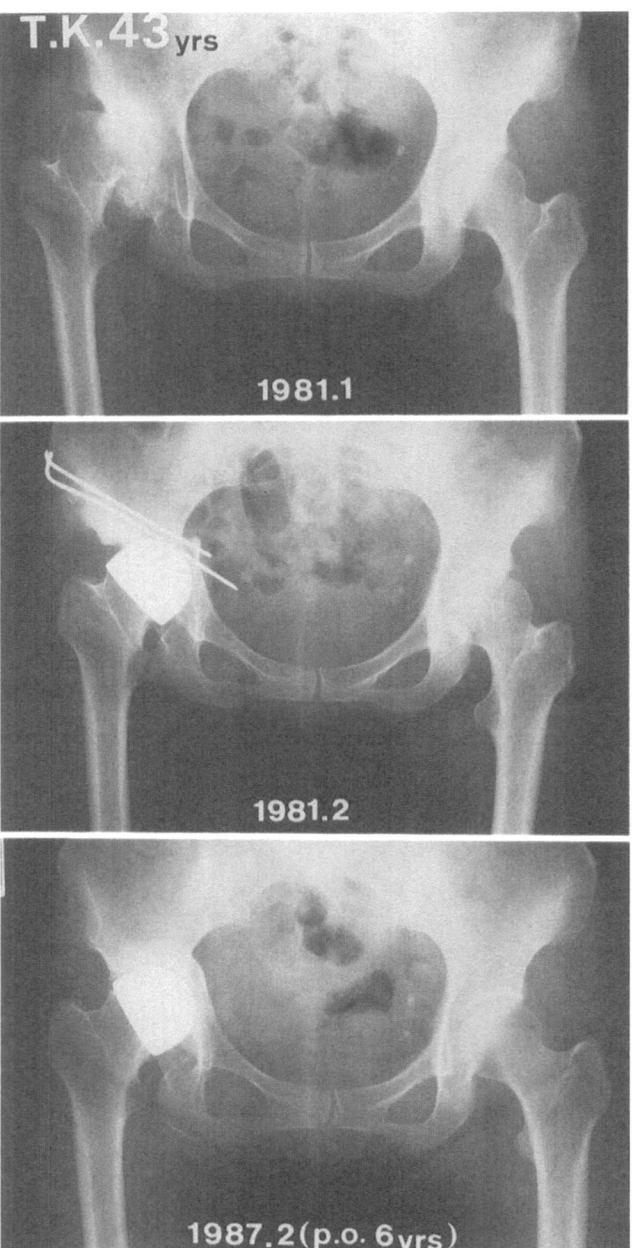

Fig. 15. Severe osteoarthrosis of the right hip (*top*) in a 43-year-old female who underwent the Chiari pelvic osteotomy combined with Cup arthroplasty (*middle*). At the 6-year follow-up (*bottom*) she had no pain

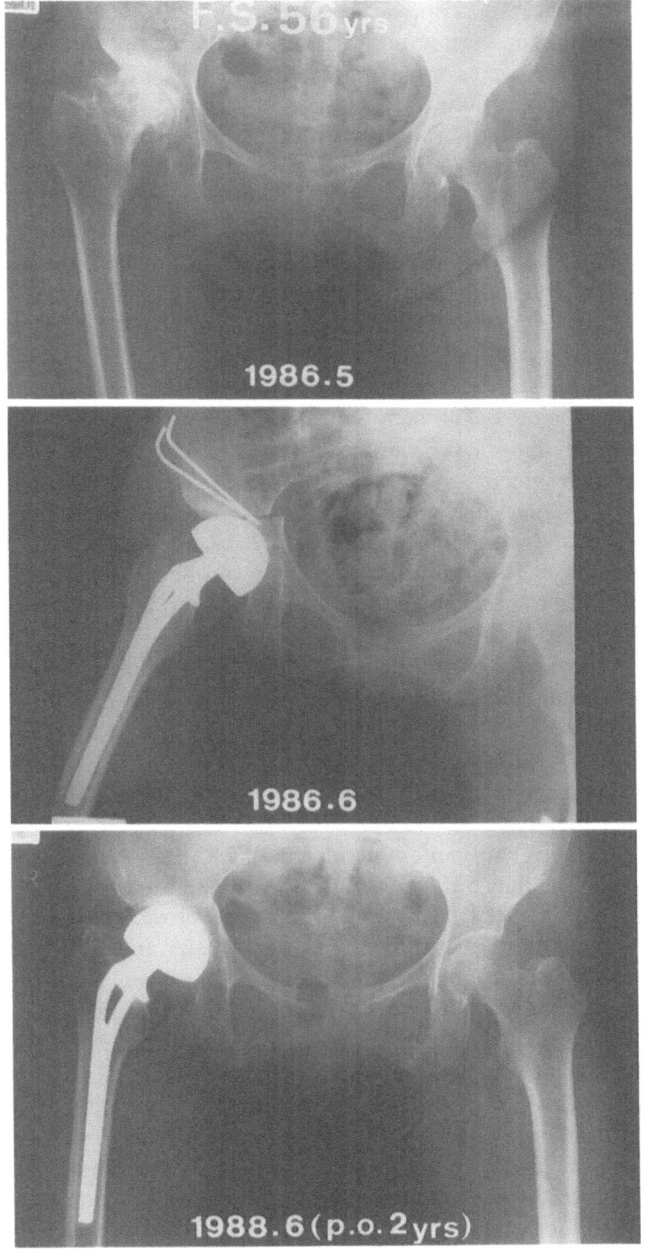

Fig. 16. Late osteoarthrosis of the right hip (*top*) in a 56-year-old female who underwent the Chiari pelvic osteotomy and bipolar femoral head replacement (*middle*). At the 2-year follow-up (*bottom*), the joint space reappeared and the subchondral sclerosis disappeared

Radiography is crucial for determining whether or not to perform the osteotomy. Before the operation, both A-P views and faux profiles are necessary. Again, indices include a Sharp's angle of greater than 55°, a CE angle of less than 10°, and a faux profile of less than 0°.

The follow-up evaluations revealed a consistent alleviation of pain, improvement of walking ability, and better ADL, except for the range of hip motion as evaluated by the JOA hip score. The total hip scores also serve as indices for patients with severely dysplastic hips.

Figures 9–12 and Table 3 compare the clinical signs with radiographic data. The scores higher than 90 points were scored by patients with Sharp's angles of less than 44° and CE angles between 30° and 40°. Faux profile anterior coverage of 20° or more was also necessary for high scores. When the osteotomy level was 4 to 8 mm from the femoral head the results were excellent. Excellent results were also achieved when the medial abductor lever arm (L1) was 60% of the lateral (L2) arm; if the ratio is more than 60%, the lateral arm should be extended by medially displacing the distal fragment.

The Chiari pelvic osteotomy is also indicated for congenital acetabular dysplasia associated with femoral neck deformity, such as in coxa valga, coxa vara, and coxa antetorta. The corrective osteotomy can be accomplished in one or two operations. We used to perform femoral osteotomy first, followed by pelvic osteotomy at the first or second sitting.

Chiari pointed out the following biomechanical disadvantages of the classical shelf operations for dysplastic acetabular roof:

1. Newly-formed acetabulum with bone grafting is intolerable to the loading of femoral head.
2. Biomechanical improvement between acetabulum and femoral head is not achieved.
3. Balance between abductor power and body weight is not improved. The ratio of the medial to the lateral arm of the abductor lever system remains unchanged.

Since his first description of the pelvic osteotomy [1], a number of orthopaedic surgeons have recognized the effectiveness and advantages of this operation. We have also postulated that there is an improvement in the congruity of the femoral head and acetabulum both in frontal and sagittal planes, widening of the weight-bearing area, and less severe loading of the extended lever arms. We feel that the method of repair of impaired osteocartilagenous tissue will be improved through better biomechanics. Despite the numerous advantages conferred, we must keep in mind the drawbacks of this osteotomy and the factors inhibiting good results. The decision process must incorporate the following factors:

1. Association of prominent coxa valga or subluxation
2. Abductor muscle weakness
3. Bilateral involvement where independent single leg stance is impossible
4. Early postoperative weight-bearing without sufficient recovery of muscle strength
5. False osteotomy level
6. Insufficient medial displacement for femoral head coverage

If these factors are absent, the long-term prognosis after this osteotomy is excellent. A unilateral prearthrosis and early osteoarthrosis of the hip with severe acetabular dysplasia in the 1st – 4th decade is the most favourable candidate for this pelvic osteotomy.

References

1. Chiari K (1956) Ergebnisse mit der Beckenosteotomie als pfannendachplastik. Z Orthop 87: 14–26
2. Chiari K (1974) Medial Displacement Osteotomy of the Pelvis. Clin Orthop 98: 55–71
3. Hirohata K, Ryo K (1979) Indication and Results of Chiari pelvic osteotomy for coxarthrosis. Clin Orthop Surg 14: 1062–1072
4. Colton CL (1972) Chiari osteotomy for acetabular dysplasia in young subjects. J Bone Joint Surg 54: B578–B589
5. Kotz R, Slaucar P (1973) Becken osteotomie und Geburt. Z Orthop 111: 797–800
6. Kotz T, Wagenbichler P (1973) Die Bedeutung der Beckenosteotomie nach Chiari für die nackfolgende Geburt Geburtu. Frauenheil K 33: 471–477

Discussion I

Sugioka (Kyushu University): I have a question for Dr. Chandler and Dr. Wilde. Your papers show a great deal of evidence for major work in revision surgery technology. In Japan, we are trying to preserve the joint, working on a more conservative approach. I think it is much more important for us to be experienced and versatile with the osteotomy, and to carry out extensive research on osteotomy. What is the future of osteotomy in the United States?

Wilde (Cleveland Clinic): I think there is definitely a place for osteotomy in the younger patient. Some of the difficult reconstructions we face now are the outcome of the total hip replacements (THR) done 8, 10, and 12 years ago; and these are serious problems. As a result we consider other procedures in younger patients that would have had a casual THR in the past. Unfortunately, there are many cases in the U.S.A. now with major bone loss from casually implanted THR some years ago.

Chandler (Harvard Medical School): I would agree entirely, but there are differences in the diseases that we are dealing with. We have far more primary osteoarthritis than in Japan where congenital dysplasia of the hip (CDH) is far commoner. Certainly, osteotomy would be the treatment of choice for the younger patient in the U.S.A. as well as in Japan.

Shiba (Kobe University): Dr. Chandler, in femoral defects due to fractures or perforation where an allograft is wired over the cortex with a cemented stem, is the original cortex not devascularized?

Chandler: The onlay grafts never completely surround the femur. We may use an entire femur as graft material but the strips have spaces between them. The onlay grafts seem to become revascularized remarkably quickly, perhaps because of the rich vascular supply of the overlying quadriceps. Also, I believe that femoral blood vessels from below and viable areas above also contribute. Whatever is happening biologically, the fractures heal readily. I believe another positive factor is the similarity of elastic modulus of the cortical onlay grafts to the patient's femur. Thus, the technique may also have a place in difficult non-unions, although we have no experience in this.

Tanaka (Kinki University): Professor Kummer, have you noted differences in bone response with different designs prostheses? For instance, femoral stems with or without a collar? Also, is there a difference if the stem has a narrow or broad taper angle?

Kummer (University of Cologne): It is very hard to say what the most desirable shape should be for an endoprosthesis because many factors are involved. Thus, if you have a long neck, greater muscular movements are produced with a smaller hip resultant force, however, the tilting moment increases so the pivot point is stressed a lot which may induce local resorption.

Alignment matters, so that a varus angle produces a greater bending moment and also greater stress at the supporting points. A valgus alignment creates less localized stress but the lever arm of the muscles is lessened making it necessary for greater muscle pull to balance the articulation; the result here is overall greater loading.

We do not know the answer yet which is why we are continuing these studies. When we have a better idea I will design a shape myself.

Tanaka: I have another question for Professor Chandler and Professor Wilde. Regarding the femoral shaft, what about the use of vascularized pedicle bone grafts?

Chandler: I have not used a vascularized pedicle graft in THR revision, but there may be a place for it. In fractures, a vascularized fibula or iliac crest has worked well. In THR revisions, the defects are often too large to be spanned by a vascularized fibula or crest and not strong enough to support weight bearing.

Wilde: I have no experience with the vascularized grafts. They have been used for avascular necrosis of the femoral head but without a demonstrated beneficial effect.

Nagaya (Nagoya University): I have experience with 1200 surgical cases, including quite a few problems of loosening and bone deficiency. From Dr. Harris's reports on the use of frozen femoral head grafts for acetabular reconstruction, we have now 55 cases with a follow-up of only a year and a half less than those of Dr. Wilde. It is my feeling that insufficient acetabular defects should be salvaged by any means and to accomplish this the use of allografts is inevitable. However, I believe that frozen bone takes more than a year to be incorporated. Therefore, I protect the patient by enforcing crutch walking for 6 months. Have you had any problems from early weight bearing?

Wilde: For the acetabulum we protect the patient for the first 3 months with crutches or a walker; then, instruct them to use a cane permanently. This is also because there are desperate problems with massive grafts and abnormal biomechanics.

Chandler: There is difference between the incorporation of cancellous bone and cortical bone. Cancellous bone, both autogenous or allograft, incorporates by bone apposition. It may actually become stronger as it is incorporated. With acetabular reconstructions we make a major effort to buttress the allografts against solid bone and hold them to that buttress with screws (the screws or fixation are not weight bearing). Since cancellous bone incorporates and becomes stronger by apposition, we encourage early weight bearing; partial weight bearing with two crutches for 6 or 8 weeks and then, on to a cane with the patient discarding the cane as soon as they can walk without pain or without a limp.

We have not had resorption of the graft with early weight bearing. In fact, I think that bone responds to the piezoelectric stimulus and becomes stronger. Thus, if bone is supported, early weight bearing is advantageous.

Cortical bone is incorporated differently with a great deal of resorption and tends to weaken as it is revascularized. However, when using the cortical bone for the femur that is on compression surfaces, such as in calcar replacement, or strut grafts on the medial side, we encourage early weight bearing. We may protect longer cortical bone on the lateral side if it is the only strength of that femur. Two cases with lateral cortical struts broke after 3–4 months as they became partially revascularized and weaker. If the stem of the component is long enough to support the bone, I think that lateral struts are all right. Thus, lateral struts used for a perforation work well.

For major allograft reconstructions we may add a long tension band plate, such as a supracondylar plate, that bypasses the junction of the allograft and the host bone.

Terayama: Professor Chandler, in some cases you used cement, and in others no cement. How do you make that decision?

Chandler: We no longer use cement on the acetabular reconstructions for almost any age, primary or revision cases. The exception may be an acetabular component without any contact with living bone using a major graft. We will accept 1/5 th contact of an uncemented acetabular component with living bone and 4/5 ths contact with allograft or autograft, if the component is well supported and well fixed.

For most femoral revisions, we prefer uncemented. In young people, with good bone (virgin) I do not use cement. The exception is elderly patients (late 70's) or physiologically elderly patients where we will cement the femur; but even in that patient, we would not cement the acetabulum. In general, the results with cement in femoral revision surgery are not as good as uncemented; loosening is common.

Terayama (Shinshu University): Dr. Chandler, in cases without cement in reconstruction of an expanded femur, what technique is used for grafting the intramedullary space?

Chandler: We use a morcelized femoral head within the medullary space for some very large proximal femoral losses within an intact rim; in one case a smaller femur allograft within a larger femur with an uncemented component.

With calcar allograft reconstruction, we insert a medial strut and fix an uncemented component into valgus, held proximally with good bone contact. If we can get the stem of the component into healthy medullary bone distally then there are good points of fixation. We then graft large defects between the two grafts with cortical strips, morcelized bone and autograft. So far they have worked well.

One problem using cement and a massive component is that the cortex is stress-shielded. If you start with a very large cavity to reconstruct with more cement and a larger prosthesis, then the next revision will leave you with almost no bone. Thus we avoid using cement in large cavities.

Torisu (Ohit University): My question is for Dr. Wilde concerning the acetabular protrusion of rheumatoid arthritis. I have experience with bipolar implants. Out of 16 cases in the past 15 years, only one case showed resorption of bone. I believe you had one case in your series with collapse. Was there any specific cause for this problem?

Wilde: No, we could not determine why that graft collapsed. In rheumatoid arthritis, however, I think it is important to do routinely bone graft for the acetabular protrusio to prevent migration of the cup into the pelvis.

Torisu: For allografts I believe it is a good idea to use a femoral head, but how do you decide when to progress to weight bearing when you cannot visualize bone union clearly on radiographs? You mentioned an average incorporation time of 11 months?

Wilde: Yes, we have experienced delayed incorporation and conventional X-ray suggested a non-union. Thus, I recommend using the three-dimensional scanner for assessment.

Iwata (Nagoya University): Dr. Kummer, when you discussed using the densitogram, you indicated that you were evaluating the stress. If the stress is increased, then bone formation is increased; when there is no stress, you have bone resorption. However, when the tissue was examined, did you see the formation of cartilage before bone formation? Can your technique distinguish between cartilage and bone?

Kummer: Regarding cartilage, appositional bone formation occurs directly from the adjacent fibrous tissue with no intermediate of cartilage. Thus, in no specimens have we seen any cartilage. The densitogram does show structural differences. Newly formed bone builds up by sheets, layer on layer, parallel to the surface. Lamellar bone has few osteons, contrary to the normal underlying bone which contains a great number of small osteons. This distinctive reorganization must be related to changes in local stresses. Lamellar bone as well as osteonal bone may not resist compressive forces but to determine this we need in vivo repeat specimens and we cannot get this information from morbid histology. I think that the lamellar bone may be secondarily replaced by osteonal bone because some osteons are seen reinforcing the bone. This will adapt it better to compressive forces.

Shiba: I think we can all use such techniques as allografting in our practice but this is still a developing area. We will need time, experience and more research before we will have better answers.

Total Condylar Knee Replacement: Late Results

ALAN H. WILDE[1]

Introduction

The total condylar knee prosthesis is a minimally constrained, stainless steel, high density polyethylene, cruciate sacrificing prosthesis which was introduced by Insall in 1974 [1] (Fig. 1). His results of a 3- to 5-year follow-up showed 93% excellent and good results in 220 cases. The infection rate was less than 2% [2]. There were no cases of loosening of the femoral or tibial component. Posterior subluxation of the tibia occurred in 1.8% of cases, largely because the distance between the cut ends of the femur and tibia were not the same in flexion and extension. There was a provision for resurfacing of the patellar articular surface with a high density, polyethylene dome-shaped prosthesis. It was demonstrated that the number of good and excellent results improved with the use of the patellar prosthesis.

The total condylar prosthesis was used with methyl methacrylate. It was a second generation prosthesis which quickly supplanted earlier, more constrained cement devices such as the Polycentric, Geometric, Guepar, and Herbert knee prostheses. Sacrifice of the cruciate ligaments and releasing the medial collateral ligament from the tibia and the lateral collateral ligament from the femur allowed correction of varus, valgus and flexion deformities without resorting to the use of a hinge prosthsis, which is undesirable because of increased rates of loosening and infection [3–5].

Later results were reported by Insall et al. in 1983 [6]. Excellent and good results were reported in 91% of 100 cases with an average follow-up of 6.6 years. The average range of motion at follow-up was 98°. Posterior subluxation of the tibia occurred in 2% of cases. Loosening of the tibial component occurred in 2%. There was no loosening of the patellar or femoral components.

Late Results of the Total Condylar Knee Prosthesis

There have been several long term reports of results with total condylar knee prosthese from several different centers. Renawat and Boachia-Adjei [7] reported results of a survivorship analysis of 90 knees with an 8- to 11-year follow-up. Results

---

[1] Department of Orthopedic Surgery, Cleveland Clinic, Cleveland, Ohio, USA

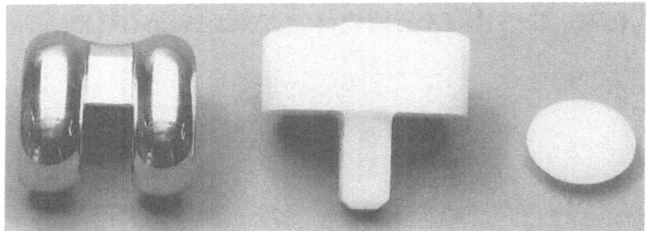

Fig. 1. Total condylar knee prosthesis

were good or excellent in 93%. There was 1 loose patellar component and 1 loose tibial component, an overall incidence of failure of 2%. Using the endpoints of survivorship as the need for revision due to septic or aseptic loosening, radiographic loosening as defined by a shift in the position of the prosthesis, or symptomatic radiolucency under the condyles of the tibia, particularly around the central peg, the survivorship was 94.1% at 11 years follow-up.

Goldberg et al. [8] reported their results in 109 knees followed an average of 9 years with a range of 7–11.5 years. The revision rate was 9%. The infection rate was 0.6%. There were excellent or good results in 64%. The rate of component loosening was 5.5%. The average range of motion was 95°. They reported a decrease in the functional knee score of an average of 7 points between the follow-up at 4 years and that at 7–11 years.

We have reported our results with the total condylar knee prosthesis at the Cleveland Clinic [9]. The first 129 consecutive prostheses performed between 1975 and 1977 were evaluated. There were 64 knees available for study with a range of 8.3–10.8 years follow-up and an average of 9.1 years follow-up. Excellent or good results were found in 77% of cases. The overall rate of tibial component loosening was 4.6%. There were no instances of femoral component loosening or patellar component loosening. None of the patients with patellar resurfacing experienced a fracture of the patella. Four revisions were performed for instability of the knee, which occurred at an incidence of 5%. There were three revisions for infection and one for patellar resurfacing. Nine of 129 knees required revision for aseptic loosening, patellar resurfacing, instability or infection. The overall incidence of failure was 6.9%.

Discussion

These late results show that the total condylar knee prosthesis is a durable implant. If the three long-term series referred to above are taken together, aseptic loosening of the prosthesis was seen in 8 of 263 prosthesis or 3%. The follow-up in these three series was from 7–11.5 years. Most of the component loosening occurred on the tibial side. No fractures of the patella occurred. The average range of motion was 97°. Posterior subluxation of the prosthesis occurred in 3.8%. There was a tendency for the results to deteriorate with time. In both the series reported by Goldberg et al. [8]

and Schurman et al. [9], the knee scores decreased with longer follow-up. After 3- to 5-year follow-up, the results showed excellent and good results in 82% and 88%, respectively. At an average follow-up of 9 years, the excellent and good results were 64% in the series reported by Goldberg et al. and 77% in the series of Schurman et al. The decline in the number of good or excellent results was attributed to advancing age and disease in other joints.

When contrasted with the long-term results of other prostheses, the total condylar prosthesis compares very favorably. The Geometric prosthesis has a reported failure rate of 18.3% after 8.5 years [10]. Freeman et al. [11] reported a failure rate of 36% after 8 or 9 years with the initial Freeman-Swanson prosthesis. In the series of Polycentric prostheses reported by Lewallen et al. [12], there was a failure rate of 34% with a follow-up of 10 years. Hamilton [13] reported a failure of 27% of University of California, Irvine (UCI) knees after 4½ years. Failure was defined as the need for an additional procedure in these series.

When the results of constrained knee prostheses are compared with the total condylar knee prosthesis, the differences are even more striking. Shindell et al. [5] reported 18 Noiles hinged knee prostheses in 1986. After an average of 32 month postoperatively, 56% had failed. Follow-up was available for more than 5 years in 17 of 18 knees. Kaufer and Matthews [14] reported 82 consecutive Spherocentric knees with an average follow-up of 4 years. The range was from 2–6 years. The infection rate was 4% and the rate of failure due to loosening was 5%. The overall re-operation rate or failure rate was 9%.

Bargar et al. [3] reported 40 Guepar and 16 Herbert prostheses after a follow-up of 2–4 years. Re-operation was required in 16% of cases due to loosening or infection. There was 1 loose prosthesis and 3 were infected. They reported that the use of either a cemented metal on metal-hinged knee replacement or a metal on polyethylene hinge-type prosthesis resulted in a relatively high incidence of failures and complications and was not the solution for treating patients with failed knee prosthesis.

Rand et al. [4] reported the results of the first 50 Kinematic rotating hinge total knee arthroplasties. The mean follow-up was 50 months, the range 29–79 months. Results in 38 knees were evaluated. There was a 16% rate of sepsis, 22% rate of patellar instability and a 6% rate of breakage of the impalant. Re-operation was required in 27 of 38 patients, a failure rate of 71%.

Ritter [15] reported the results of 30 Herbert total knee arthroplasties after a 3-year follow-up. Seven of 29 were subsequently replaced for metallic synovitis and an additional knee was replaced for infection. The re-operation rate was 27% due to synovitis or infection. In addition, Murray et al. [16] reported a 14% incidence of fracture of the femoral component of the prosthesis in a series of 23 Herbert knee replacements. The fractures occurred as early as 5 months postoperatively.

While the total condylar knee prosthesis cannot be successfully utilized for all conditions of the knee, a number of the knees treated by hinge-type prosthesis can be successfully treated by the total condylar knee prosthesis. Furthermore, when the total condylar knee prosthesis is compared to a newer porous-coated knee prosthesis such as the porous-coated anatomical (PCA) knee, there was a revision rate of 7.8% with the PCA knee reported by Hungerford [17] after a follow-up of 4–6 years. All in all, the total condylar prosthesis seems to be one of the most durable implants available at this time for the treatment of knee diseases.

Bibliography

1. Insall JN (1981) Technique of total knee replacement. In: The American Academy of Orthopaedic Surgeons. Instructional course lectures. vol 30. CV Mosby, St. Louis, pp 324–334
2. Insall JN, Scott WN, Ranawat CS (1979) The total condylar knee prosthesis. A report of 220 cases. J Bone Joint Surg 61: A173–A180
3. Bargar NL, Cracchiolo A, Amstutz HC (1980) Results with the constrained total knee prosthesis in treating severely disabled patients and patients with failed total knee replacements. J Bone Joint Surg 62: A504–A512
4. Rand JA, Chao EYS, Stauffer RN (1987) Kinematic rotating hinge total knee arthroplasty. J Bone Joint Surg 69: A489–A497
5. Shindell R, Neumann R, Connolly JF, Jardon OM (1986) Evaluation of Noiles hinged knee prosthesis. J Bone Joint Surg 68: A579–A585
6. Insall JN, Hood RW, Flawn LB, Sullivan DJ (1983) The total condylar knee prosthesis in gonarthrosis. A five to nine year fellow-up of the first one hundred consecutive replacements. J Bone Joint Surg 65: A619–A628
7. Ranawat CS, Boachie-Adjei O (1987) Survivorship analysis and results of total condylar knee arthroplasty. Orthop Trans 11: 66
8. Goldberg VM, Figgie MP, Figgie HE III, Heiple KG (1988) Use of a total condylar knee prosthesis for treatment of osteo-arthritis and rheumatoid arthritis: Long-term result. J Bone Joint Surg 70: A802–A811
9. Schurman JR, Borden LS, Wilde AH (1987) Long term results of total condylar knee prosthesis. Orthop Trans 11: 433
10. Riley D, Woodyard JE (1985) Long term results of geomedic total knee replacement. J Bone Joint Surg 67(4): B548–B550
11. Freeman MAR, Todd RC, Bamert P, Day WH (1978) ICLH arthroplasty of the knee: 1968–1977. J Bone Joint Surg 60: B339–B344
12. Lewallen DC, Bryan RS, Peterson LFA (1984) Polycentric total knee arthroplasty: A 10-year follow-up study. J Bone Joint Surg 66: A1211–A1218
13. Hamilton LR (1982) UCI total knee replacement: A follow-up study. J Bone Joint Surg 64: A740–A744
14. Kaufer H, Matthews LS (1981) Spherocentric arthroplasty of the knee. J Bone Joint Surg 63: A545–A559
15. Ritter MA (1977) The Herbert total knee replacement: A longer than 3-year follow-up. Clin Orthop 129: 232–235
16. Murray RG, Wilde AH, Werner F, Foster D (1977) Herbert total knee prosthesis. J Bone Joint Surg 59: A1026–A1032
17. Hungerford DS, Krackow KA (1987) Five year follow up of a cementless total knee replacement, Orthop Trans 11:442
18. Borden LS, Heyne T, Belhobek G, Marks KE, Stulberg BN, Wilde AH (1982) Total condylar prosthesis. Orthop Clin North Am 13: 123–130

Principles of Alignment in Primary and Revision Knee Replacement

T. Derek V. Cooke[1]

Introduction

Most agree that current knee replacement surgery is directed toward the resurfacing of the joint with reconstitution of physiological features, and most current designs employ anatomically shaped femoral components. All systems are geared toward the restoration of the load-bearing axis (LBA) as a line of force (body weight) passing through the hip to the ankle through the centre of the knee. Most procedures are aimed to reconstitute the joint line but opinions differ on the coronal orientation of the joint [1-3]. Most systems also advocate balance of the soft tissues [1, 3, 4].

Loosening of total knee replacement (TKR) has been closely associated with non-anatomic designs [4, 5]. Loosening and poor kinematics occur with a poor fit of the components and loosening is enhanced by poor fixation. However, loosening and poor kinematics are most often related to malplacement and malalignment of the prosthetic parts [1, 3-5]. The problems of malalignment and malplacement are under the surgeon's control and it is thus critical that precise measures are taken to prevent these problems. More problems occur with varus malalignment and severe inward obliquity of the bearing surfaces, predisposing subluxation. Subluxation has a greater tendency to occur in prostheses with the least constraint.

What Is Ideal Alignment?

There are few reports in the literature on this subject [6]. The data from my department, derived from a study of healthy young adults (25 males and 25 females) using standardized radiographs [7], revealed no sex differences in angular geometry and a mean for the LBA that passed through the knee 0.3° away from its centre (Fig. 1). While this overall alignment varied little, the orientation of the joint line (respective rotation of the femoral condyles and tibial plateau to the hip and ankle), varied in a reciprocal manner, such as to maintain the LBA close to zero[8]. Thus, in the healthy young adult a valgus rotation of the distal femur (to the hip) was usually compensated for by a varus rotation of the tibial plateau (to the ankle), and vice

---

[1] Clinical Mechanics Group, Queen's University, Kingston, Ontario, Canada

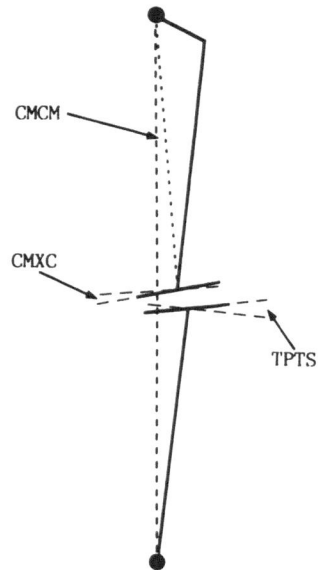

	MEAN	ST DEV
CMCM	0.3	1.2
CMXC	+3.8	2.1
TPTS	-3.3	2.2

>90°

Fig. 1. Physiological alignment in young adults. *CMCM*, Capitomidcondylar-capitomidmalleola; *CMXC*, Capito-midcondylar-transcondylar; *TPTS*, tibial plateau-tibial shaft angles

versa, maintaining the LBA at zero. The joint line had a mean inward obliquity to the LBA of nearly 4° more than a right angle.

If this alignment is "normal," where should the implant be placed? In osteoarthritics, joint line obliquity is increased and a wide range of deformities is encountered. Hungerford et al. [2] attempted to restore the level of the joint line and inclined it 3° inward to the LBA. They reason that a "physiological" orientation is best for functional restoration of the knee. Bargren et al. [1], Insall et al. [3], and many other reports, including the report of our group [9], recommend *no* inward slant, i.e., an orientation of the implant joint line at right angles to the LBA.

This alignment of the joint is rationalized on the basis that it is more stable in the coronal plane than an inward slant and better able to resist the outward buckling and shear forces applied by the body in the single leg stance phase of gait. Current implants do not reconstruct the congruity formed by the femur articulating with both menisci with their conforming submeniscal tibial geometry. The only resistance given to lateral shear stresses in a prosthesis is the upward slant of the tibial eminence and to a lesser extent, any "cupping" provided by the tibial surface. Thus, current implants are less conforming than the real knee and have a greater tendency for coronal subluxation. This tendency may be lessened if the joint line approaches a right angle to the applied load.

Other reasons for loosening include debris of polyethylene, due to wear, creating inflammatory membranous changes capable of inducing bone resorbtion [10]. If carbon is in the wear particles (hard and brittle) the reaction may be magnified. Another potent mechanism for polyethylene wear debris is the presence of intra-articular loose beads, which may have come away from a poorly scintered porous-coated implant [10]. Deficient bone, as may be seen in rheumatoid arthritis and magnified by the use of steroids, may have added risks for implant subsidence. Finally, infection, when it occurs, will also promote loosening.

Minimal Surgical Error

The vital overall principle is to lessen surgical error. To do this, machining technology has been applied to TKR using a frame in which the knee is aligned and onto which a tri-axial saw is mounted to cut the bone [9]. The femur and tibia are separately aligned in the frame on functional axes of each bone and held with transfixion pins [9, 11].

The second principle, implicit to using resurfacing components, is to position each new surface in direct relationship to the ligaments. Thus soft tissue rebalancing (releasing contracture and shortening overly long ligaments), must be undertaken and then the implant is positioned to these ligaments (Fig. 2a, b). This measure preserves bone stock and will optimize kinematics. It must be emphasized *not* to use bone parts of the joint as a guide to location of the implant since these surfaces are arthritic, deformed, abnormal and are being replaced. Rather, the author advocates that the location of the implant is in direct relation to the ligamentous structures (the posterior cruciate and collateral ligament origins) (Fig. 2a).

The Principles in Revision Arthroplasty

These principles are essentially the same as in primary knee arthroplasty. Alignment is critical. However, there is also a new important problem because loosening produces bone destruction and bone stock must be re-established.

The lost bone may be restored by the use of autografts or allografts. Autogenous bone is preferable where available. But in revision the only source may be the iliac crest. Femoral head or other sources of cancellous bone from frozen allografts may then be used. It is important to restore as much of the bone as is feasible, filling in any remaining "gap" by the use of "deeper" prostheses (thicker femoral and/or tibial components may be needed). The second added problem in revision is stability. Rarely in revision are the cruciates well preserved and collateral structures may also be deficient. Stemmed implants have a role in this situation as do implants with more stable geometry (built in restraint). Thus, cruciate sacrificing designs with posterior stabilizers and occasionally implants with hinged rotational design features may be necessary. The following illustrative cases outline these concepts.

Case Report

Case 1. This 70-year-old female patient had a University of California, Irvine (UCI) prosthesis which loosened (Fig. 3a) and was subsequently replaced with a condylar-type prosthesis with an allograft on the medial side (Fig. 3b). The implant however, was aligned in varus. Bone scans showed activity in the graft (incorporation) but also

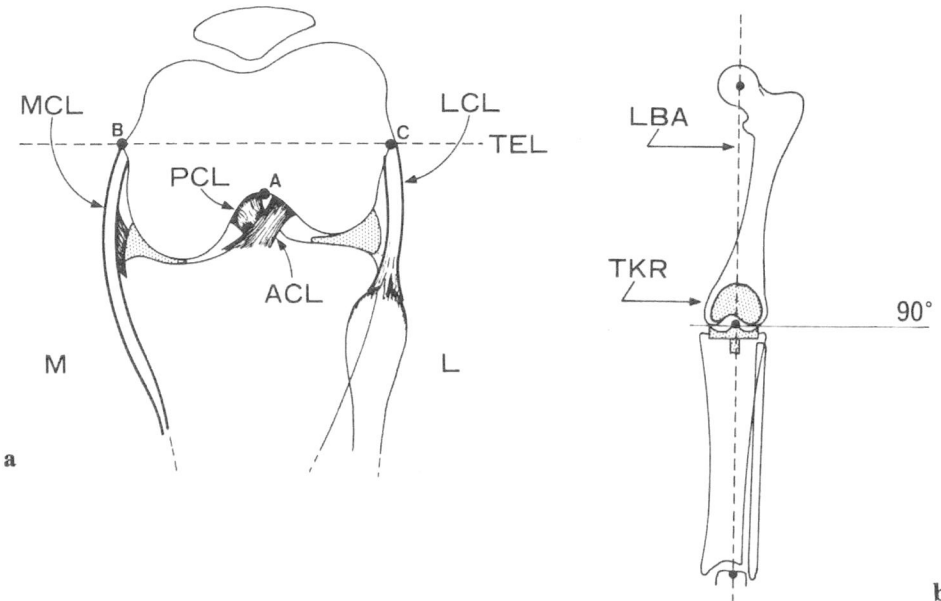

Fig. 2 a,b. Alignment of TKR. **a** In 90° flexion *TKR* insertion is best centered to ligament origins (*A*). Posterior cruciate ligament (*PCL*); neutrally rotated to, medial collateral ligament (*MCL*), (*B*) and lateral collateral (*LCL*), (*C*) on the transepicondylar line (*TEL*). **b** Aim for reconstitution of the joint line square to load-bearing axis (*LBA*)

changes in the bone beneath the prosthesis (Fig. 3c). Further loosening occurred requiring revision to a rotating hinged-type implant (Fig. 3d).

Bone defects may be central, or more commonly peripheral. In a primary TKR, where the defect is tibial, the bone graft may be taken from the femoral condyles, and sometimes taken as a horizontal slab from the opposite side of the tibia. Grafts are fixed using small cancellous screws countersunk into the bone. Once the bone stock is restored it is critical to cut the load-bearing ends square to the functional axes of each bone (Fig. 2b). This ensures that the graft and bone are exposed to evenly disposed compressive forces. An accurate fit of the graft is also important.

Case 2. This case was a revision of a previous double osteotomy which resulted in considerable valgus of the tibia (Fig. 4a). A square cut in the remaining tibia would entail excessive bone loss of the proximal denser load-bearing region. Thus, a slab of bone was cut from the lateral proximal tibial plateau which provided the donor material to be transferred medially to a square cut site and held with screws (Fig. 4b).

Case 3. In this case 2 revisions were required. This 72-year-old male had a failed geomedic prosthesis which was revised. The design features of this prosthesis impose high shear stresses at the bone-cement interface under load. At revision low-grade

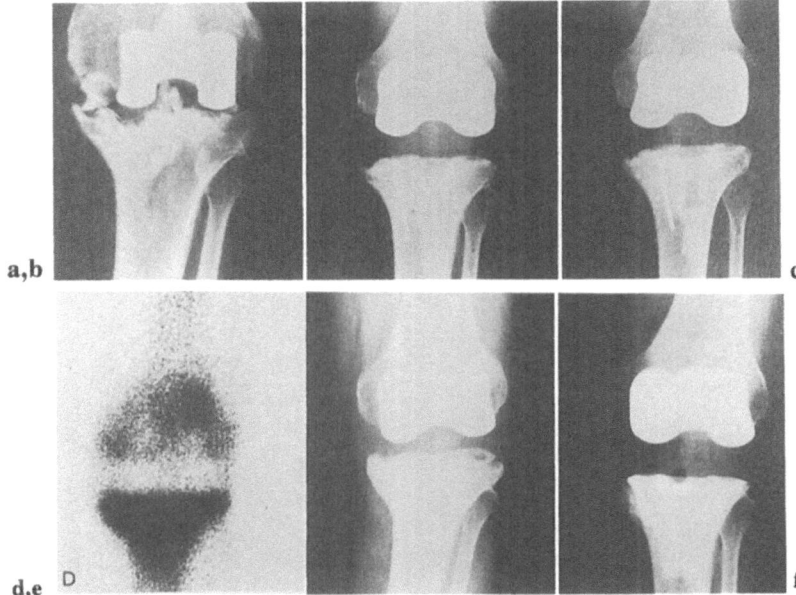

Fig. 3 a-d. Sequence of views in revision of a loose Irvine TKR. **a** Loose Irvine prosthesis. **b** Reconstituted with graft but in varus. **c** Revision still in varus. **d** Bone scan indicating further loosening **e** Further loosing. **f** Final revision square to LBA

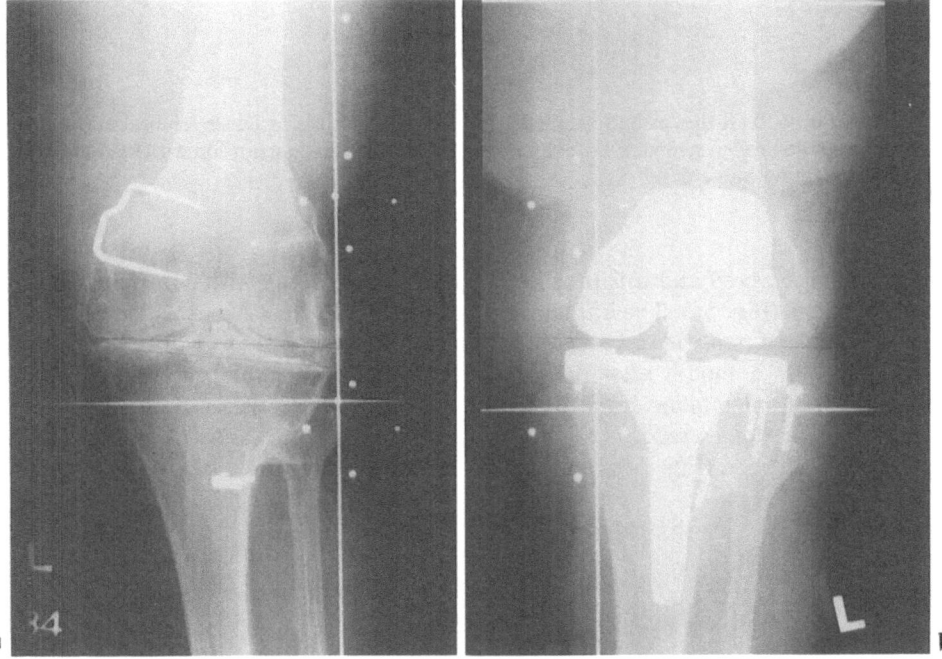

Fig. 4 a,b. Revision double osteotomy. **a** Excessive tibial valgus. **b** Postoperative graft cut square from the lateral side and screwed medially into square cut slot

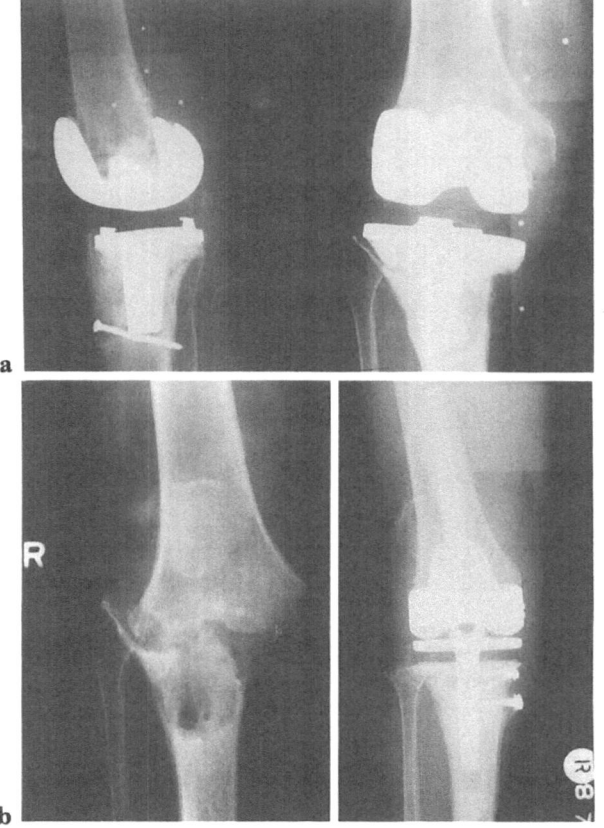

Fig. 5 a-c. Loose TKR due to bad geometry and secondary sepsis. **a** Loose femoral and tibial prostheses (note broken screw). **b** Defect following removal. **c** Reconstitution with medial bone graft and rotating hinge design

sepsis was discovered and this prosthesis proceeded to loosen with subsidance into the tibial bone (Fig. 5a). The implant was removed with extensive debridement and the patient was fitted with a cast. Massive proximal bone was lost from the medial tibia (Fig. 5b). A month after debridement, aspiration and biopsy cultures were negative; tibial bone taken from the high lateral side was transferred medially and fixed with cancellous screws. A rotating hinge implant was necessary to make up the remaining lost bone (Fig. 5c). This patient is now 5 years post surgery and doing well.

Discussion

The results of revision surgery are seldom as good as the primary replacement. As seen from these examples and from the literature, revisions have a high failure incidence. The principles for alignment used in revision surgery are the same as in primary surgery with the added need for reconstitution of bone and potential requirement for more stable stemmed implants. The surgeon's aim must be not to revise, and since alignment and mal-position are so strongly implicated in loosening, the surgeon must be precise and accurate in primary implant placement. This fact supports the use of machining principles in TKR.

Acknowledgment. The author acknowledges the valuable support of the Clinical Mechanics Group members in the technology described in this paper.

References

1. Bargren JH, Blaka JD, Freeman MAR (1983) Alignment in total knee arthroplasty: Correlated biomechanical and clinical observations. Clin Orthop 173: 178–183
2. Hungerford DS,.Kenna RV, Krackow KA (1982) The porous coated anatomic total knee. Orthop Clin North Am 13: 103
3. Insall J, Tria AJ, Scott WN (1979) The total condylar knee prosthesis: the first 5 years. Clin Orthop 145: 68–77
4. Lotke PA Ecker ML (1977) Influence of positioning of prosthesis in total knee replacement. J Bone Joint Surg 59: A77–A79
5. Kagan, AII (1977) II Mechanical causes of loosening in knee joint replacement. J Biomech 10: 387–391
6. Moreland JR, Bassett LW, Hanker GJ (1987) Radiographic analysis of the axial alignment of the lower extremity. J Bone Joint Surg 69-A, No. 5: 745
7. Wevers HW, Siv DW, Cooke TDV (1982) A quantitative method of assessing malalignment and joint space loss of the human knee. J Biomed Eng 4: 319–324.
8. Nguyen C, Bryant JT, Cooke TDV, Chow D (1988) Alignment and geometry of the normal knee in stance. The Canadian Orthopaedic Association 43rd Annual Meeting Proceedings, Ottawa, Ontario, Canada
9. Cooke TDV, Saunders G, Siu D, Yoshioka Y, Wevers H (1985) Universal bone cutting device for precision knee replacement arthroplasty and osteotomy. J Biomed Eng 7: 45–50
10. Wevers HW Cooke TDV (1987) Bead loosening in porous metal coated implants: A case study. Clin Materials 2: 67–74
11. Yoshioka Y, Sui D, Cooke TDV (1987) Anatomy and functional axes of the femur. J Bone Joint Surg 69-A, No. 6: 873

Discussion II

Kurosaka (Kobe University): Dr. Wilde, as you know cementless prostheses are being used with the expectation of greater longevity, what is your feeling on this question?

Wilde (Cleveland Clinic): Our long-term study of cemented total knee replacement (TKR) is comparable to the results from the Hospital for Special Surgery. Both show a very similar and acceptable outcome — a failure or loosening rate of 10% over 9 years. The defects of the total condylar design, including the problems of subluxation, alignment, and limited flexion, have largely been corrected with the posterior stabilized prosthesis. I am aware of a number of loosenings in cementless knees within the first 2–3 years. There are no long-term results. So, I currently prefer to use a cemented knee, confident that this knee is going to last a long time.

Cooke (Queen's University, Ontario): This is an important question. I agree with Professor Wilde that the old standard is now the total condylar cemented knee and the results are really very good. Thus, we should not switch easily to another system without evidence that this will be better.

The evidence of Dr. L. Ryd from Sweden, using stereophotogrammatory, is that the uncemented porous-coated anatomical (PCA) tibial component subsides. There is very little available data to suggest bone ingrowth at the tibia. Ryd indicated that studies of the Miller-Gallante knee, in which the tibial component is strongly screwed into the bone, showed little micromovement.

Another problem of uncemented designs using beads is that the beads may break away, end up in the joint and produce high density polyetheylene (HDPE) wear particles. These create inflammation and potentiate loosening. The final problem, on which Professor Kummer might comment, is the relationship to stress shielding. If the implant does become biologically fixed, then this heavy, rigid component may result in marked cancellous bone change. Interestingly, when we cement, we may give a wider stress distribution to the bone and different patterns of bone remodelling.

Kummer (University of Cologne): I fully agree with Dr. Cooke. The most important problem facing us is how to reach relatively equal stress distribution between the endoprosthesis and the bone. This occurs when the resultant force of the new joint falls into the center of the weight-bearing surface. Secondly, the force should be distributed at 90° to the surface lessening shearing stresses. Thirdly, and perhaps most importantly, is the nature of the intermediate between the metal and the bone; cement may play a very important role in shock absorbtion and in a better distribution of force.

Yamamoto (Matsuyama Red Cross Hospital): Over the past 8 years I have used cementless TKR in nearly 600 cases. Only 3% showed aseptic loosening. The majority of loosened cases were found on the femoral side — few occurred on the tibial side. Why, in the case of cementless prosthesis, does the loosening occur at the femur, whereas, with cement this happens at the tibia?

Wilde: That is a good question. I have always assumed that the loosening of a cemented prosthesis on the tibial side was due to the greater stresses, particularly in rotation through the tibia. No loosening on the femoral side is a common observation with cemented prostheses. I think this is due to the geometric fit of the prosthesis on the bone cuts; it provides stronger resistance to shear stresses. It is not clear why a cementless prosthesis loosens on the femoral side, because the same principles of a good geometric fit should be operational.

Kummer: I believe that aseptic loosening is generally seen at the femur. This would be expected from the biomechanical point of view. Computer simulation of knee kinematics show that the resultant of the knee joint in stance, for reasons of equilibrium, must always fall rectangularly to the tibial surface. Only during movement does it wander anteriorly or posteriorly. The change in direction and location of the resultant force however, is relatively greater on the femur. Thus, at the surface, shear forces may appear.

Tateishi (Hyogo Medical University): I use a ceramic cemented prosthesis, however, in my experience, the tibial side subsides most. It is my opinion that when we are dealing with rheumatoid arthritis (RA), with the osteoporosis, cement should be used.

Yoshiya (Kobe University): As Dr. Cooke mentioned, this is an important issue that needs a lot of research. However, we must move on to the next issue regarding the preservation or sacrifice of the posterior cruciate ligament (PCL) during TKR.

Wilde: The use of this prosthesis or the posterior stabilized, condylar prosthesis requires the excision of both cruciate ligaments; the advantage being the capacity to correct virtually any deformity. Also only one prosthesis is needed for stability, not a series in different configuration. Soft tissue releases, that I described, are needed to correct severe deformity which when using a cruciate-sparing prosthesis is often very difficult.

Cooke: The prediction that a relatively more constrained design, such as that used in total condylar — posterior stabilized prosthesis, would result in a high incidence of loosening has not been borne out by the clinical results. The choice of different designs, from constrained to less constrained patterns, has not been shown to be a major advantage yet.

On the other hand, if we are aiming towards normalizing kinematics of the knee, then the knee that is lacking the cruciates is biomechanically inferior. The evidence to support this comes from gait and stair climbing analyses done by Andriacchi from Rush Presbyterian Center in Chicago. The cruciate retained showed much better function, especially in stair climbing. Also, when considering the long-term outcome in terms of function of the knee in younger patients, I suspect that major advantages will be seen with cruciate-sparing prostheses.

Our experience bears out aspects that Dr. Wilde has mentioned. Deformity and kinematics are more difficult to correct with a less constrained prosthesis that retains the cruciates; balancing the soft tissues is even more important as well as more difficult. In every severe cases, not only must the tight side be released but also the lax side may need tightening. This requirement has occurred most often in a severe valgus deformed knee. Finally, I feel we are still a long way from developing an ideal prosthesis which should also include functioning meniscal elements.

Yoshino (Tokyo): I sacrifice the PCL in all cases. The reason is to preserve as much good subchondral bone of the tibia by performing very limited bone resection. When you then compare the level of the joint postoperatively, it is higher. When you retain the PCL, the joint space is constrained and flexion is inhibited. The second reason is as described by Dr. Wilde; balancing the collateral ligaments in the PCL retained knee is difficult. Valgus deformity is the most difficult to obtain optimal balance. Regarding problems of cruciate resection, in my experience, I have not had any that are severe problems. I would like to mention another feature which is very interesting. When revising TKR's, I have noticed that the postero-capsule forms a condensed thickening in the PCL area. In vivo the PCL is very important and even when sacrificed the body shows some capability of making a similar structure.

Wilde: Regarding any problems with sacrificing the PCL, I would have to say yes there are problems, when the prosthesis does not substitute for the resected ligament. We have four cases of tibio-femoral instability in the total condylar knee.

As to your second question about a complex forming in the posterior capsule that is like the PCL, I have not seen that.

Cooke: In respect to the PCL limiting flexion. I am not convinced that the PCL is at fault. I think many factors play a role. In our instrumentation technique, all the bone cuts are made in flexion and the ligaments are balanced before the bone cuts are made. The retained PCL does not prevent further flexion.

I find your report of neo-PCL being formed very interesting. Our observations in some TKR that were re-explored was that the body had made meniscal-like structures that filled the spaces between the prosthetic margins. If appears that the body is telling us it prefers to have a ligament and a meniscus. So, perhaps, the optimum is to preserve these elements.

I have been performing PCA knee for a number of years. While it is disturbing to sacrifice the PCL, often a very long deep posterior band remains. We found 20% of the knees had a posterior sag in flexion, but this did not seem to be important clinically. Our 5-year study on PCA knee has shown that no revision is necessary.

Kinoshita (Tokushima University): I have more than 10 years experience in sacrificing PCL. As already mentioned by the speakers, the correct alignment is very important. When we sacrifice PCL, the posterior sagging is related to the lack of sufficient tension in the remaining soft tissues. The tension gap must be filled; a total condylar extra thick tibial component may be used to do this. Do you use spacers?

Wilde: Metal spacers are used to check the gap in flexion which should be the same as that in extension. We use the thickness of the tibial plateau that will accommodate this.

Cooke: In principle, we use the same.

Okamoto (Yokohama City University): I would like to ask this question of Dr. Cooke. You mentioned that the cruciates should be preserved when possible. At our center we have many RA patients. These patients seldom have an anterior cruciate ligament (ACL) — the PCL is usually intact. When we hesitate to sacrifice PCL we use the kinematic anterior joint type. Our results show good stability and alignment which has been maintained.

Kurosaka: This opinion differs from that of Dr. Yoshino who felt that sacrifice of the PCL did not influence the stability. What happens in the case of a minimally constrained prosthesis?

Yoshino: In our cases of TKR the stability is maintained by the soft tissues, even though we sacrifice the PCL.

Kurosaka: So, the latero-medial ligaments compensate for that. Is that your opinion?

Yoshino: Yes.

Yamamoto: For more than ten years, I have sacrificed both ligaments, ACL and PCL and I agree with Dr. Yoshino. In TKR, in order to restore the stability of soft tissues, alignment must be correct, including rotational deformity.

Kurosaka: We are dealing with a very difficult issue which needs more study. Dr. Cooke, do you have a brief comment?

Cooke: I am interested that those two comments advocating resection of PCL, so as to stabilize the knee. Surely, when you take the ligaments out, you are making the knee more unstable. So, that it is quite logical when you remove the cruciate ligaments, you *must* provide some other kind of change in the nature, the shape or thickness, of the prosthesis to replace them. Most designs incorporate some feature in their geometry, which replaces the cruciate ligament. The most critical factor is to prevent posterior subluxation. This point has been clearly made by Dr. Wilde. Thus, I suspect that the geometry features of both the Yoshino type of prosthesis and the Yamomoto prosthesis under load become stable. It does not make sense however, to say that you are making the knee more stable by taking the cruciates out. What is clear is that when you take the cruciates out, you correct the deformity more easily. Now, the question is, will the long-term kinematic result be better with or without the cruciates? It does not appear that the knee without the cruciates and with a more restrained shape has a high incidence of loosening.

Yoshino: The prosthesis I am using is a non-constraint type tibial component; the surfaces are laterally flat.

Kummer: The whole kinematics of the knee are totally changed if you remove one of the cruciate ligaments. The whole process of movement depends strongly on the position, the morphological shape, the structure, and the length of the cruciate ligaments. The lack of cruciate ligament however, can be compensated for, certainly for a while, by other structures. For example, by the menisci, by other soft tissues, and to some extent by muscular forces. The question is, how long will this compensation last?

Kurosaka: This is a difficult issue which will have to be clarified from further research and long-term studies. Dr. Cooke has emphasized the importance of accurate instrumentation for bone cutting and many doctors agree with this. Yesterday, Dr. Cooke presented this topic with data of a new jig. The jig is very precise, but it looks very complicated. How long does it take to set up the saw jig prior to surgery; how long does it take to cut the bones?

Cooke: These are important questions. It takes about 15–20 minutes set-up (non-tourniquet) time. In terms of the actual surgery, when we started with the earlier models, it often took between 2 and 3 hours. The operative time is down now with the Mark III Questor Jig and comparable with other instrumentation, usually less than 2 hours.

Watanabe (Watanabe Orthopedic Hospital): I would like to pose a question. When there is extreme varus malalignment and a major release is undertaken and there is still 5° varus, should the medial collateral ligament be sectioned to correct it?

Wilde: That is a definite occurence — an insufficient release. Usually, it is a semimembranosis that has not been released enough, or one that has not gone far enough distally to release the pes anserinus and the superficial collateral. You may need to release completely around the upper end of the tibia and posteriorly, so that the tibia is dislocated anterior to the femur. It is then much easier to release the semimembranosis and the posterior capsular attachment on the tibia. You should then correct all the varus deformity. If there is a bowed shaft of the tibia that may need a different approach.

Watanabe: If there is severe bowing of the tibial shaft do you need to think about an osteotomy?

Cooke: Our morphologic studies show that varus deformity occurs mainly at the upper end of the tibia. When the varus deformity is proximal I correct it with a knee replacement and medial release. If the varus deformity is very significant distally, then, I think there will be kinematic imbalance, unless you do an osteotomy beforehand.

Koshino (Yokohama City University): I want to ask about alignment. Dr. Wilde, your results showed an average alignment of 3° valgus. However, 7° is the average. Were you aiming for 7° and the result was 3° or did you aim for 3° from the beginning? I would also like to ask about the HS knee score. How man of the 87 knees scored 90 or greater?

Wilde: In the clinical ratings, 77% were good or excellent — in the same range as a hospital for special surgery rating. Regarding the desired valgus, I agree we should aim for 5°-7° of valgus. We are not satisfied with our end result (mean of 3° valgus) — a number of cases were still in varus. The reasons were the following: 1) These were the first cases of knee replacement. 2) There were five surgeons involved. 3) The instrumentation was not optional.

Yoshino: In order to achieve good alignment, you must balance the soft tissue. When this is balanced, what is the ideal orientation? Dr. Cooke recommends a 90° position to the load-bearing axis (LBA). I agree with him. From my experience the 90° position for balancing soft tissue can be obtained in all cases. In the extended position you do not achieve equal balance.

Kinoshita: To have an accurate bone cut, one must have an accurate knowledge of thhe femoral axis and tibia. I have used various instruments in the past, but I think a good method to define the axis is the use of an intramedullary (IM) rod. Cutting guides can be attached to the axial guide to a cut at 175° for FTA (femoro-tibial angle) or 172°. But in Japan, a 9–10 mm IM rod is optimal. If the patient is large, an 11 mm may be used.

Kurosaka: Finally we would like to discuss revision surgery. At the rheumatoid arthritis session, infection after TKR was a major topic. I would like to concentrate on late infections. Can one re-implant in revision surgery?

Wilde: For infected total knee replacements, we advise a 2-stage operation. The first stage is to remove the infected prosthesis and cement, debride all damaged tissue, and take cultures frm the cement membrane. We then insert an antibiotic cement spacer. The antibiotics chosen are based on the organism obtained by aspiration before surgery. We then re-aspirate the knee weekly for 3 weeks. If the cultures are sterile, then at 4 weeks we undertake re-implantation. The results have been very satisfying. We have had 2 failures in nearly 20 cases. One case. One case was *Clostridium perfringens* and a mixed infection, in which we ended up fusing the knee. Another failure was due to Morganella which is resistant to antibiotic treatment. However, cases infected with *Staphylococcus epidermidis* and gram-negative organism sensitive to antibiotics were successful.

Biomechanics of the Ankle

ROGER A. MANN[1]

Introduction

The biomechanics of the ankle joint cannot be considered as an isolated entity but, as stated by the late V. T. Inman, should be thought of as the "Joints of the Ankle". The ankle joint undergoes dorsiflexion and plantar flexion during gait and transmits rotation in the horizontal plane. The transverse rotation which crosses the ankle joint is translated by the subtalar joint into inversion and eversion. This coordinated function of the ankle joint and subtalar joint has been likened to a universal joint. The motion of the subtalar joint in turn controls the transverse tarsal joint (talonavicular and calcaneocuboid joint), which functions as a locking and unlocking mechanism of the midfoot. The interdependency of these joints on one another is why this complex is considered the "Joints of the Ankle."

Ankle Joint Orientation

The orientation of the ankle joint is illustrated in Fig. 1. The axis of the ankle joint is 20°–30° externally rotated in relation to the knee joint but the foot is aligned internally in relation to the ankle. The tibial plafond is parallel to the ground but the axis of the ankle joint, as measured from the tips of the malleoli, is deviated medially.

   The articular surface of the talus does not represent a section from a cylinder but rather one from a cone whose apex is directed medially. The apical angle is about 26°, although there is considerable variation (Fig. 2).

Ankle Motion

Ankle motion which occurs in the sagittal plane is dorsiflexion and plantar flexion. Figure 3 demonstrates that at the time of heel strike plantar flexion is occurring at the ankle joint, following which there is progressive dorsiflexion until approximately 40% of the walking cycle, when plantar flexion begins once again, and it terminates at the time of toe-off, when dorsiflexion once again begins.

[1] Department of Orthopedic Surgery, University of California School of Medicine, Oakland, California, USA

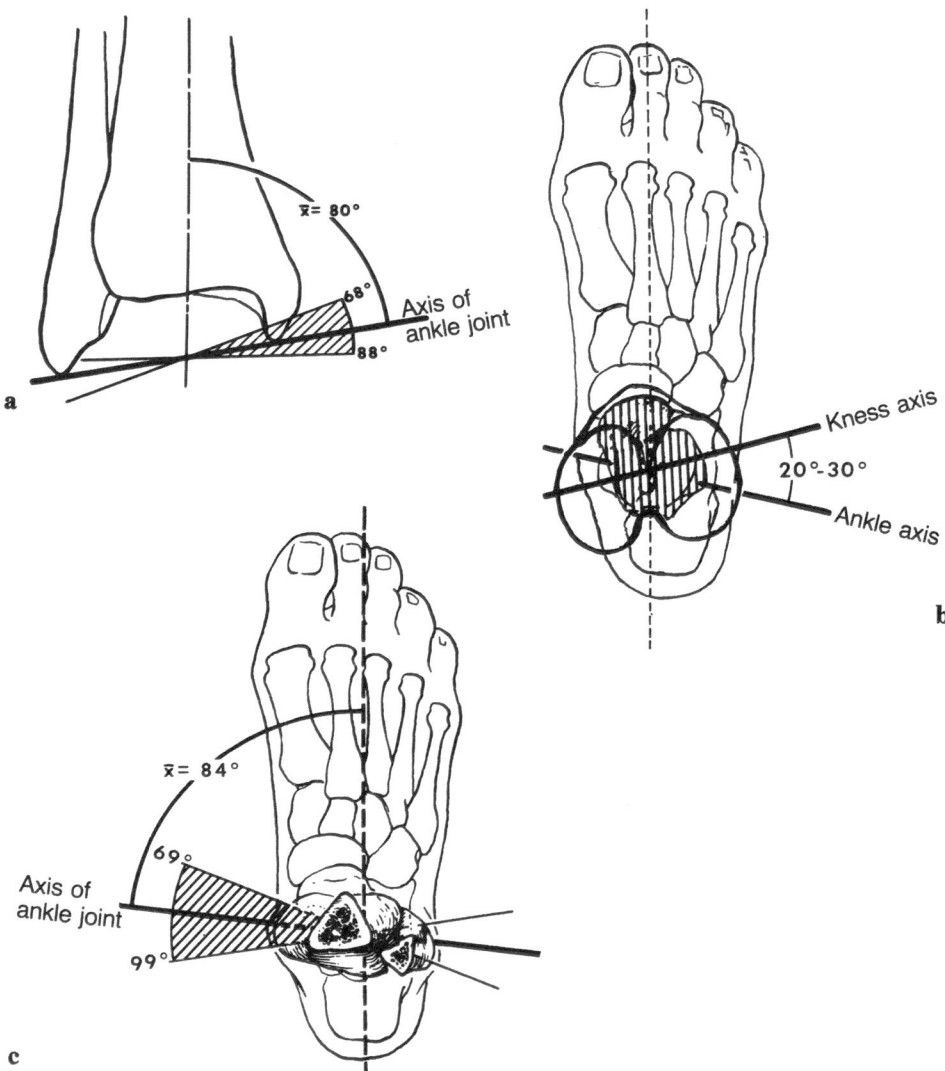

Fig. 1 a-c. a Variations in the frontal axis of the *ankle joint.* **b** Relationship of the *knee* and *ankle axes.* **c** Relationship of the ankle axis of the foot. From [3]

This ankle joint motion is controlled by the muscles of the leg. The anterior tibial group is thought of as a dorsiflexor of the ankle joint, and the gastrocsoleus group as plantar flexors. When one carefully analyzes Fig. 3, it can be observed that the anterior tibial muscle group (which includes the extensors) is active at heel strike when plantar flexion is occurring. What we are observing is that the anterior tibial muscle group is controlling plantar flexion of the ankle joint at the time of heel strike, and after dorsiflexion of the ankle joint has been initiated the muscle group is

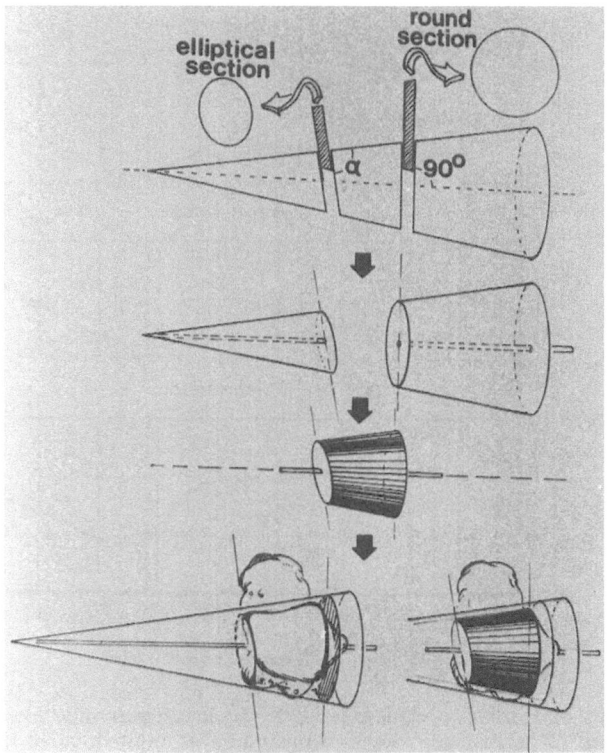

Fig. 2. The articular surface of the talus is a section from a cone whose apex is directed medially. From [2]

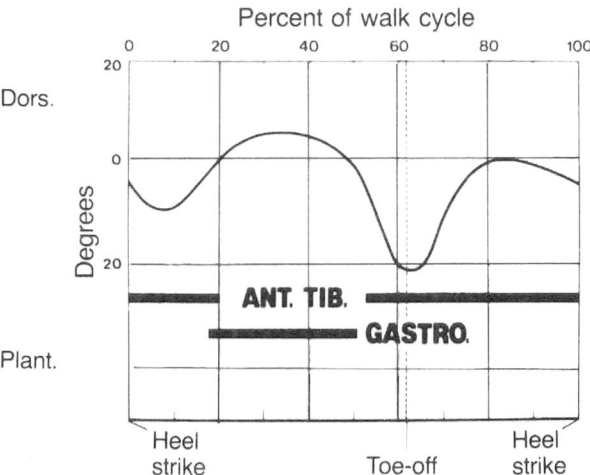

Fig. 3. The range of motion of the ankle joint along with the phasic activity of the anterior tibial (*ANT. TIB.*) muscle representing the anterior compartment and of the gastrocsoleus (*GASTRO*) muscle rerpesenting the posterior compartment

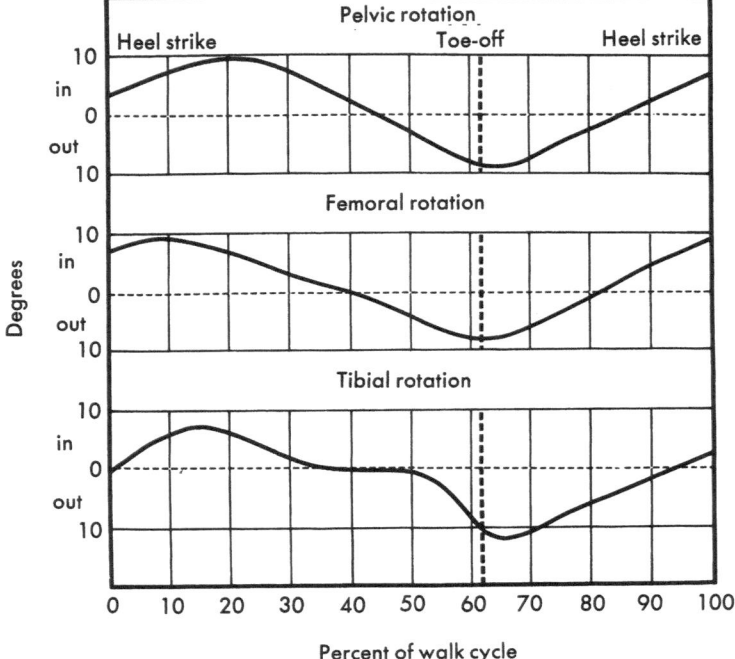

Fig. 4. Transverse plane rotation in the lower extremity. Inward rotation is occurring at the time of heel strike, reaches a maximum at approximately 15% of the cycle when outward rotation begins, which reaches a maximum at toe-off, when inward rotation resumes. From [4]

no longer active. The muscle group then becomes active just prior to toe-off, when dorsiflexion of the ankle resumes, and maintains its activity through the opposite heel strike. If this muscle group is not functional, due to an affliction such as polio-myelitis or discogenic disease, the patient will develop a foot drop during the swing phase — which would be compensated for by excessive knee flexion during the swing phase, and a foot slap at initial ground contact, because there is no muscle to control the initial planter flexion. The function of the gastrocsoleus muscle initially is to control the progressive dorsiflexion of the ankle joint during the first half of the stance phase. By controlling forward movement of the tibia over the foot which is fixed to the ground, it secondarily promotes stability of the knee joint as the body moves over the stance leg. At approximately 40% of the walking cycle, plantar flexion begins at the ankle joint, mediated by the gastrocsoleus muscle group.

It is interesting to note, however, that the muscle function ceases prior to full plantar flexion. If the gastrocsoleus muscle were nonfunctioning, the effect on the gait cycle would be loss of stability at the ankle joint, which would result in the ankle joint going into marked dorsiflexion during the midstance phase, and secondarily there would be some instability at the knee joint.

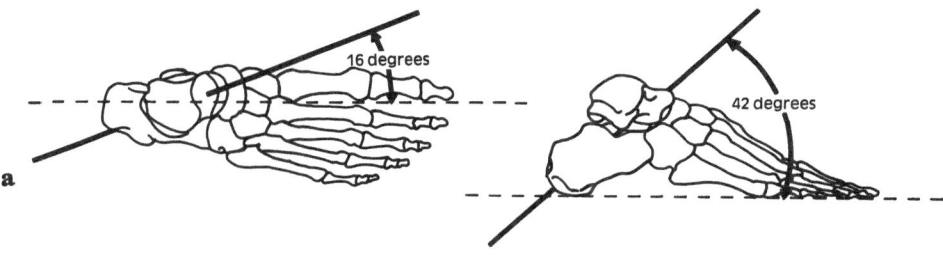

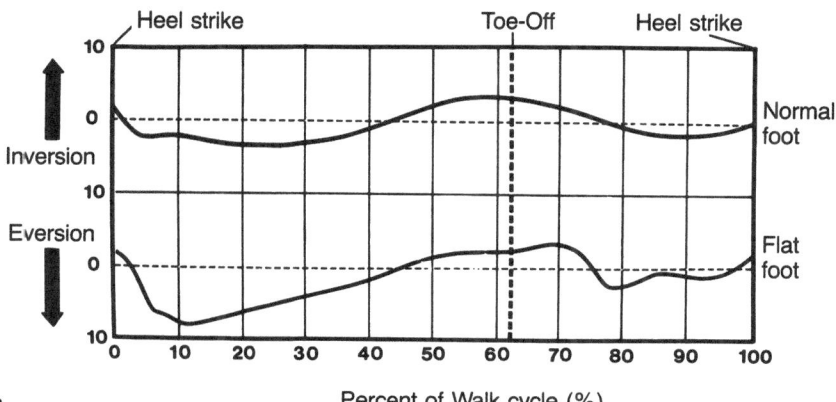

Fig. 5 a,b. a Axes of the subtalar joint. **b** Rotation of the subtalar joint. At the time of heel strike eversion is occurring which reaches a maximum at 15% of the cycle, at which time progressive inversion begins until the time of toe-off, when eversion resumes. Note that the degree of rotation is greater in an individual with a flat foot. From [5]

Transverse Plane Motion

The transverse plane motion which occurs in the lower extremity is illustrated in Fig. 4. It is noted that there is inward rotation occurring in the pelvis, femur and tibia at the time of heel strike, which reaches its peak at approximately 15% of the walking cycle. Following this there is progressive outward rotation occurring until the time of heel strike, when inward rotation once again resumes.

The effect of this transverse rotation which is translated by the ankle joint to the talus is that it results in movement of the subtalar joint. The subtalar joint is illustrated in Fig. 5a, and its axis is such that it functions as a mitered hinge. This permits movement in the (tibia) above to be translated into movement of the calcaneus below. The rotation in the subtalar joint, as noted in Fig. 5b, demonstrates that at time of heel strike there is eversion occurring until foot flat is achieved at about 15% of the cycle, when progressive inversion begins until the time of toe-off, when eversion resumes. This inversion and eversion is mediated across the transverse tarsal joint, which in turn provides stability to the longitudinal arch of the foot.

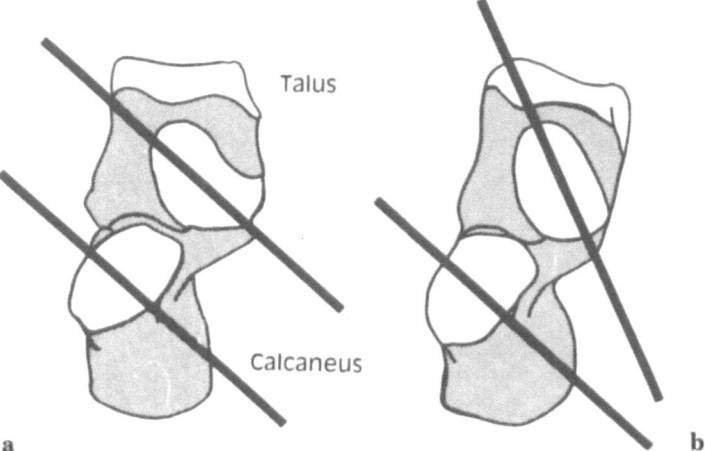

Fig. 6 a,b. Relationship of the axes of the transverse tarsal joint. **a** When the calcaneus is in everted position, the axes are parallel, giving rise to a flexible midfoot. **b** When the calcaneus is in an inverted position, the axes are nonparallel, which gives rise to stability of the midfoot

The transverse tarsal joint, as demonstrated in Fig. 6, consists of the talonavicular and calcaneocuboid joints. With inversion and eversion of the subtalar joint the calcaneus moves beneath the tibia, which brings about change in the axis system which affects the stability of the longitudinal arch of the foot. When the calaneus is in an everted position the axis system is parallel, providing less stability, whereas when the calcaneus is in an inverted position the axis system is nonparallel, giving rise to increased stability to the longitudinal arch.

Rotation of the Tibia

The model depicted in Fig. 7 demonstrates the events occurring about the joints of the ankle during internal and external rotation of the tibia. Figs. 7a and c demonstrate that inward rotation of the tibia results in the movement being transmitted across the ankle joint and translated in the subtalar joint to inversion. This is turn locks the transverse tarsal joint, establishing a rigid longitudinal arch. Figs. 7b and d demonstrate that outward rotation of the tibia is transmitted across the ankle joint and translated by the subtalar joint to eversion of the calcaneus and unlocking of the longitudinal arch, giving rise to a flexible foot.

At the time of initial ground contact the weight of the body against the foot brings about eversion of the calcaneus, which results in the internal rotation of the lower extremity above. The degree of internal rotation, I believe, is mediated by the overall posture of the foot; namely, a flat foot will have more rotation and a cavus foot less rotation. Muscle force per se does not play a significant role in the degree of internal rotation at the time of heel strike but rather it is the configuration of the foot that determines the magnitude. The rotation reaches a maximum at the time of foot flat

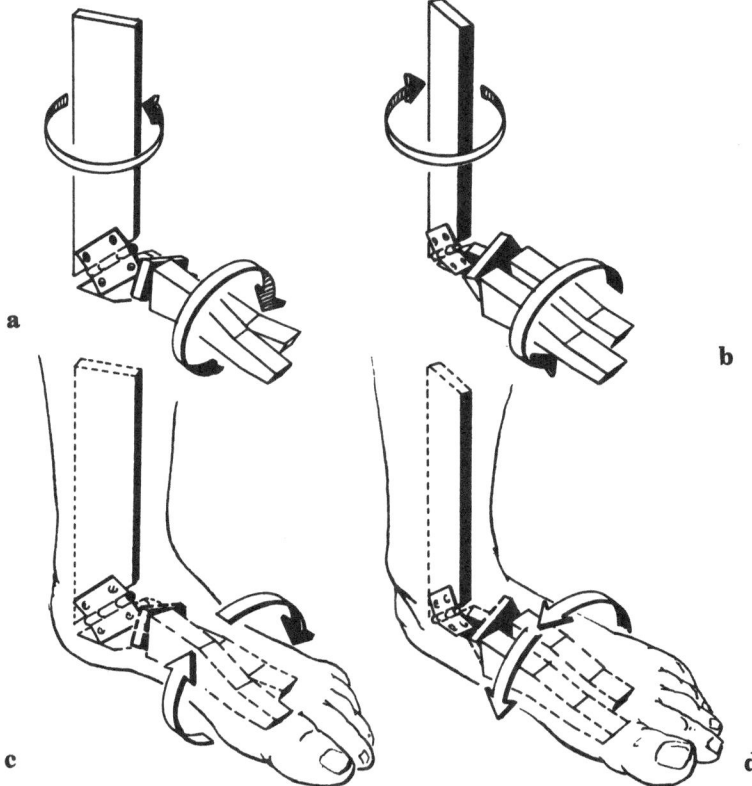

Fig. 7 a-d. and **b** represent a stick figure of the tibia articulated via the subtalar joint to the transverse tarsal joint and the medial and lateral rays of the foot. **a** and **c** represent inward rotation of the tibia, which results in inversion of the calcaneus and locking of the midtarsal joint. **b** and **d** represent inward rotation of the tibia, which results in eversion of the subtalar joint and unlocking of the transverse tarsal joint and hence the midfoot. From [2]

when, due to the movement of the contralateral limb, progressive external rotation is brought about. This external rotation is mediated from the outward rotation of the pelvis, which acts as a crank-type mechanism against the femur, which in turn transmits this rotation across the knee and ankle joint, where it is translated by the subtalar joint to inversion. It is through this basic mechanism that stability of the longitudinal arch is achieved during normal gait.

Ankle Ligaments

The ligaments about the ankle are demonstrated in Fig. 8. The calcaneofibular ligament is parallel to the axis of the subtalar joint. When the ankle is in plantar flexion the anterior talofibular ligament is in line with the fibula, thereby providing stability

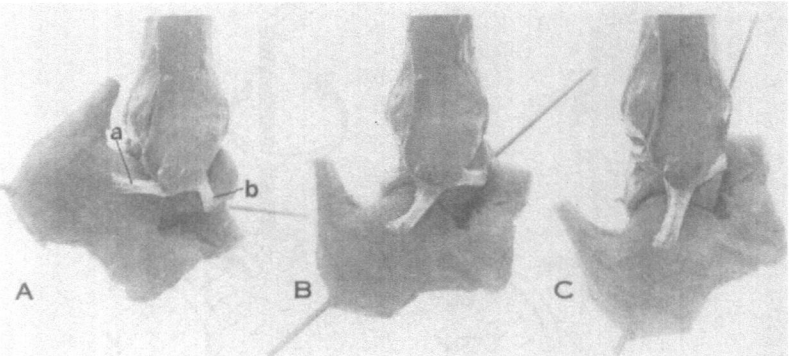

Fig. 8 A-C. The ligaments about the ankle. **A** The calcaneofibular ligament (*a*) is parallel to the axis of the subtalar joint. **B** In plantar flexion, the anterior talofibular ligament is in line with the fibular. **C** In dorsiflexion, the calcaneofibular ligament is in line with the fibula. From [3]

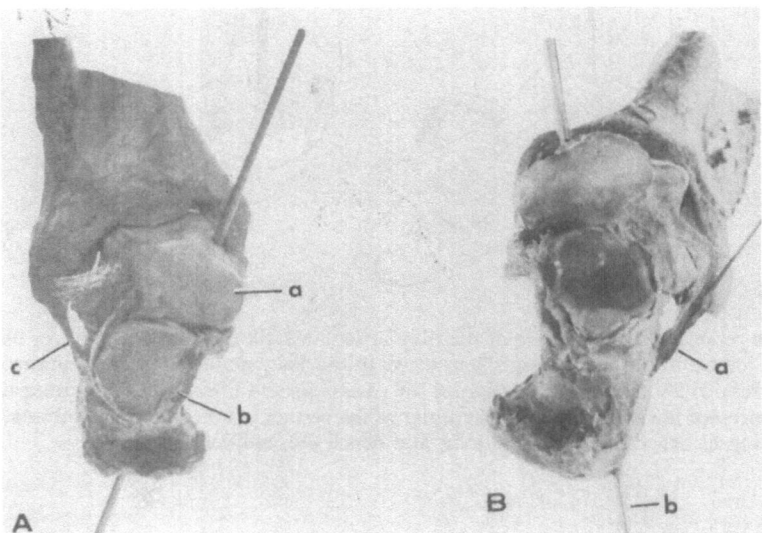

Fig. 9 A,B. Relationship of the ankel ligaments and the subtalar joint. **A** The axis of the subtalar joint is marked with a Steinmann pin. The calcaneofibular ligament is labelled *c*. **B** A Steinman pin is inserted into the calcaneofibular ligament, labelled *a*. Note the V-shaped configuration between the line of the calcaneofibular ligament and the axis of the subtalar joint. From [2]

to the ankle joint. In dorsiflexion, the calcaneofibular ligament is in line with the fibula, providing lateral stability. From a clinical standpoint, the anterior talofibular ligament is more prone to injury since the ankle joint is in a plantar flexed position when the inversion stress is applied. If the ankle joint was in a dorsiflexed position, such as if one were to step in a hole, the calcaneofibular ligament could be torn.

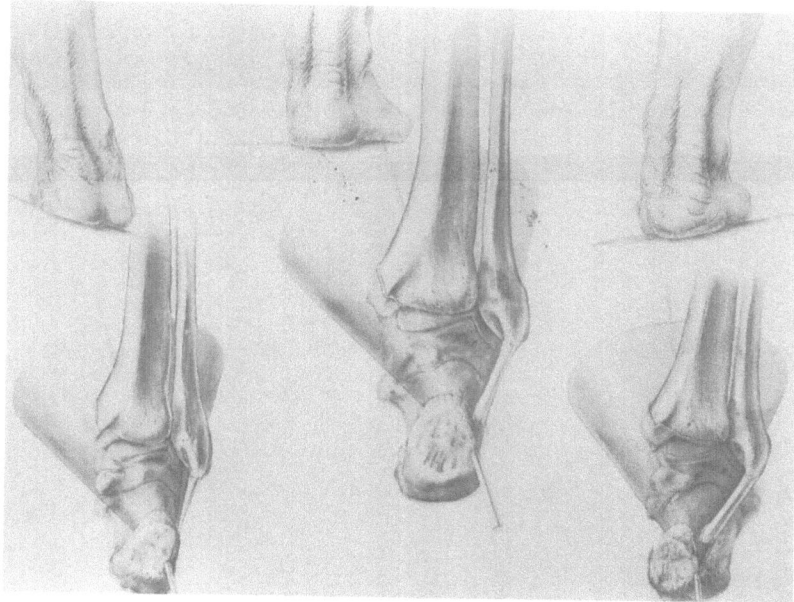

Fig. 10. As the subtalar joint moves from inversion (*left*) to eversion (*right*), the calcaneofibular ligament rotatesw around the back of the ankle joint. From [2]

The relationship of the ankle ligaments to the subtalar joint is extremely important. In Fig. 9a, b, note the V-shaped configuration between the line of the calcaneofibular ligament and the axis of the subtalar joint. When the subtalar joint moves from inversion to eversion, as demonstrated in Fig. 10, we observe that the calcaneofibular ligament rotates around the back of the ankle joint. This rotation of the calcaneofibular ligament behind the ankle is very critical in permitting full motion to occur in both the ankle and subtalar joints. If this ligament is reconstructed incorrectly, then, since the calcaneofibular ligament spans two joints, it will restrict either the ankle and/or the subtalar joint movement. This is why whenever the calcaneofibular ligamant is reconstructed it should be along its anatomic axis and not at a right angle to it, as is carried out with the Watson-Jones type of repair.

Bibliography

1. Elfman H (1960) The transverse tarsal joint and its control. Clin Orthop 16: 41
2. Inman VT (1976) The joints of the ankle. Williams and Wilkins, Baltimore
3. Isman RE, Inman VT (1969) Anthropometric studies of the human foot and ankle. Bull Prosthet Res 10–11: 97
4. Levens AS, Inman VT, Blosser JA (1948) Transverse rotation of the segments of the lower extremity in locomotion. J Bone Joint Surg 30: A859
5. Wright DG, Desai ME, Henderson BS (1964) Action of the subtalar and ankle-joint complex during the stance phase of walking. J Bone Joint Surg 46: A361

Current Status of Total Ankle Replacement

RICHARD N. STAUFFER[1]

Summary. Clinical experience with total ankle replacement (TAR) has been disappointing overall. However, satisfactory results in rheumatoid patients and elderly patients with post-traumatic osteoarthritis (OA) (who are less physically active) have been achieved. Knowledge gained from further study of the mechanical function of the normal, diseased and prosthetic ankle joint should allow development of improved TAR design for better function and durability.

Introduction

The clinical results of total ankle replacements (TAR) have been disapointing. Although the need for TAR is less than that for replacements for diseases of the hip or the knee, there are a number of problems of the ankle which are optimally treated by replacement. These include rheumatoid arthritis (RA), secondary post-traumatic OA and rarely, primary OA. There are only two treatment options available when conservative treatment has failed: an arthrodesis or TAR. Fusion remains the procedure of choice for most cases and yields a satisfactory result in the majority, but dissatisfaction is not uncommon (about 20%). A number of complications can occur, including delayed union, nonunion or malunion (40%). An average of 5.5 months of immobilization is required to achieve union. A pseudarthrosis rate of approximately 20% has been reported and the initial clinical results are poor in 30% of cases. Further, OA in the subtalar and midtarsal joints is reported to develop in about half of the cases within 8–10 years [1–5].

The kinematic study of the tibio-talar (ankle) joint indicates the motion needed at the ankle during normal level walking averages some 26°. But to climb stairs, 35° of motion are needed and descending requires 55°. During walking we found no single point of rotation (to indicate pure sliding of the talus within the mortise) but rather constantly changing instantaneous centers of rotation (Fig. 1). Thus, both rolling and sliding motion occurs during gait. However, the variation in the elipsoid pattern, described by the instantaneous centers of rotation, was small enough for practical purposes to consider the ankle as a pin joint.

---

[1] Orthopedic Surgery, Mayo Clinic, Rochester, Minnesota, USA

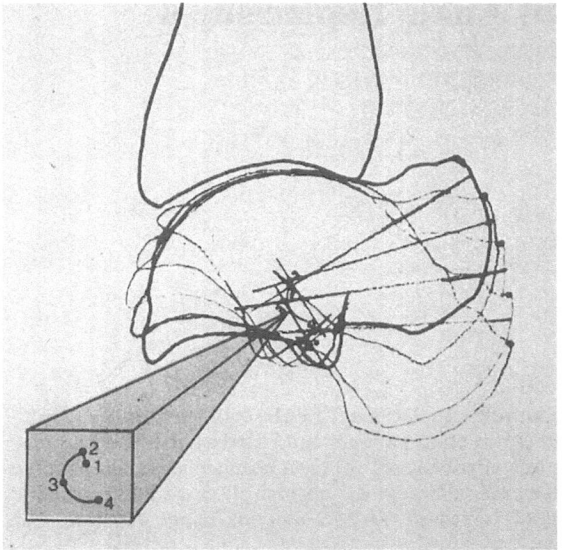

Fig. 1. Instantaneous center of rotation of the ankle from full dorsiflexion to full plantarflexion

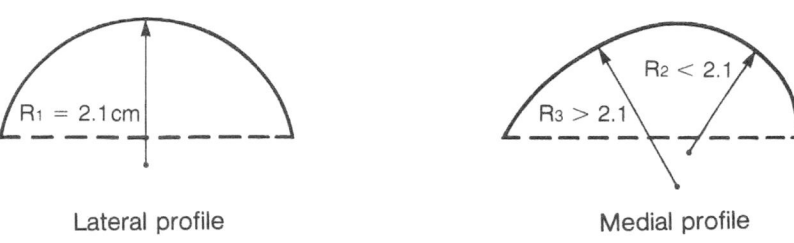

Lateral profile   Medial profile

Fig. 2. Radii of curvature of medial and lateral aspects of the talus

The talus shows a difference in radii of curvature between lateral and medial sides (Fig. 2). The talus has been described as a truncated cone, but in reality it is more complex. On the lateral side of the talus there is a uniform radius of curvature of approximately 2.1 cm. On the medial side of the talus, the radius of curvature of the posterior portion is more than 2.1 cm, while the radius of the anterior portion is less than 2.1 cm. This denotes varying axes for planter flexion and dorsiflexion, which confers some 12° of rotation of the talus within the ankle joint mortise from full plantar flexion to full dorsiflexion.

The forces acting across the ankle were analyzed using a high speed movie camera mounted on a walkway at the level of the ankle joint, plus the use of a piezo-electric cell force plate. Using a computer program the anterior tibial tendon force, the Achilles' tendon force, the compressive or "normal" and the tangential or shearing forces about the ankle were calculated. The results of this study have been published [5], and are shown in Fig. 3. The compressive force across the ankle increased to approximately five times body weight toward the end of the stance phase of gait (80% of the stance phase). The shear torque force reached a maximum of approxi-

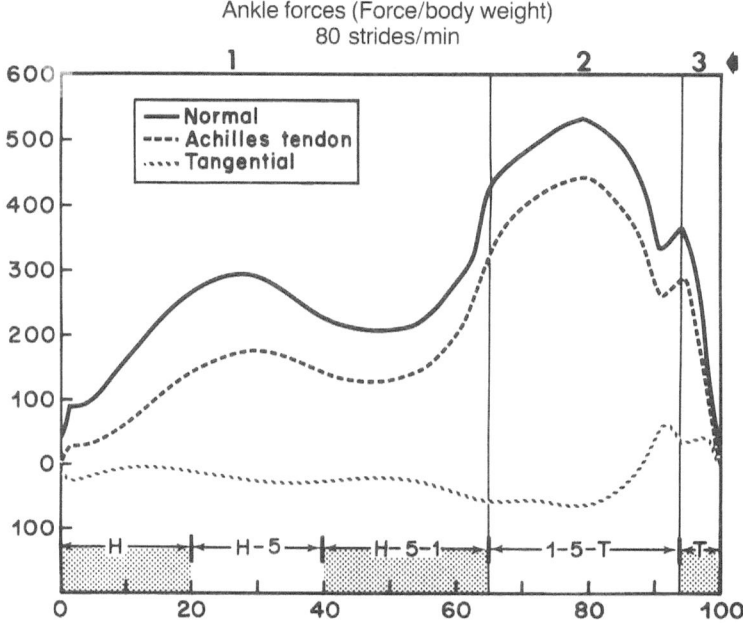

Fig. 3. Results of a two-dimensional, quasi-static loading study of the normal ankle joint during gait

mately 60% of body weight, at about 80% of the stance phase. This compressive load was much greater than was anticipated and is apparently greater than forces at the hip or the knee. As this was a two-dimensional study, a three-dimensional analysis might show even higher loads. The surface area of the ankle joint is about 10 cm². Thus, if a 70-kg man bears five times his body weight through the joint it would result in a total force of 350 kg, and if evenly distributed, 39 kg per square centimeter. The compression yield strength of ultra-high density polyethylene is 225 kg per square centimeter (six times the amount of stress that one may anticipate across a prosthetic ankle.) Our studies suggested that the ankle joint is stable and kinematically rather simple, but bears tremendous compressive loads easily because of its large surface area. This may explain why the ankle joint is rarely subject to primary OA.

The design of the current Mayo TAR, developed in 1974, embodies a polyethylene tibial component and a vitallium talar component. The radius of curvature of the bearing surface is 2.1 cm, with an area of 9cm². The device is constrained to permit motion only in one plane (sagittal); lips of the polyethylene component prevent rotation (Fig. 4). a smaller model of this device which is reduced 20% in all dimensions is also available. The clinical experience with the Mayo TAR extends from 1974 to 1981, permitting a follow-up of at least 4 years [7]. The numbers of RA cases have remained stable each year but the post-traumatic cases have decreased, as we have noted more problems with the TAR in these cases. Some very difficult problems, such as pseudarthrosis or previous ankle fusions, were operated on early in this

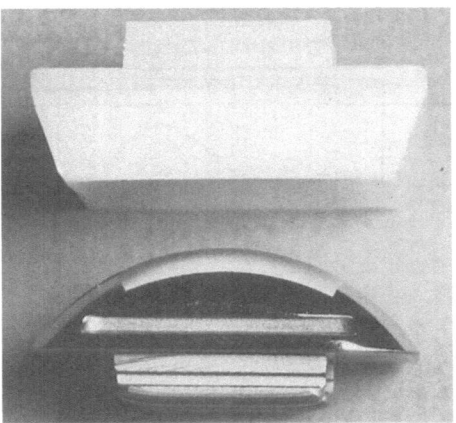

Fig. 4. Lateral view of original Mayo Total Ankle Prosthesis

series. Added factors indicating a need for TAR are bilateral ankle joint disease and degeneration of the mid-tarsal or subtalar joints. In case example, a 70-year-old male had post-traumatic OA involving both ankles (Fig. 5a, b) and bilateral total ankle arthroplasties were performed (Fig. 6a, b).

It was realized with time that patient selection is extremely important. The criteria used in assessing the results were: excellent: complete pain relief, improved ambulation and motion; good: no more than mild pain, ambulatory capacity and functional range of motion improved; fair: mild to moderate pain, no improvement in ambulation, loss of ankle motion; poor: needing subsequent surgery (revision) or severe pain. Combining the excellent and good results yielded a satisfactory rating of 74% of 187 cases; 26% were unsatisfactory (fair or poor). Stratification of results according to age and diagnosis was done. In patients with RA, 83% achieved a satisfactory result, but in OA and post-traumatic cases, only 63% were satisfactory. The data for post-traumatic OA (mean age 57 years) were disappointing but 76% of cases over 60 years showed satisfactory results. Patients with RA were younger (51.4 years) and their results showed little decline over the follow-up period.

The range of motion achieved by TAR was disappointing; preoperative patients had a mean of only 21° and postoperatively the mean motion increased to only 25.7°. For level walking this may be adequate, but it is not sufficient to ascend or descend stairs normally (more than 50° optimal). Complications included deep infection in 2.7% (all were RA patients taking steroids) and persistent pain. Painful loosening required fusion in 8%. Fusion was achieved in all but one of the 15 cases, using a compression distraction technique [8]. Talo-fibular impingement was a rather common problem which occurred early. About five-sixths of the compression load on the ankle acts through the tibio-talar joint and about one-sixth through the oblique talo-fibular joint. The Mayo TAR does not address the replacement of the talo-fibular joint and thus continued pain from impingement in the talo-fibular joint occurred in about 20%. Occasionally, additional surgery was performed to decompress the impinging surfaces at the talo-fibular joint. Excision of this joint, to avoid impingement, should be a routine part of the TAR procedure.

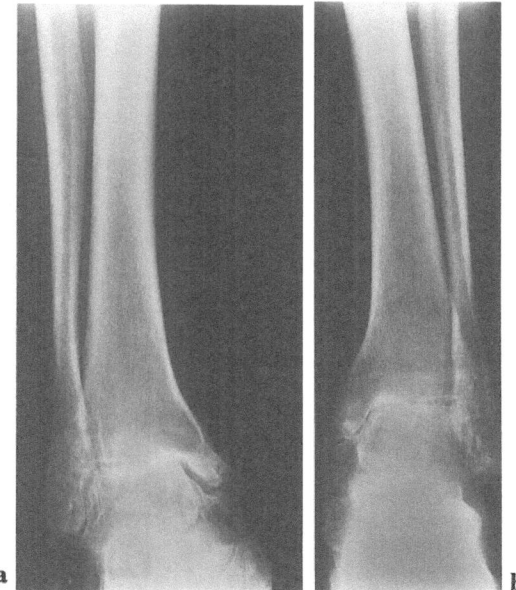

Fig. 5 a,b. Anteroposterior roentgenograms of a 70-year-old man with osteoarthritis of both ankles (**a** left, **b** right)

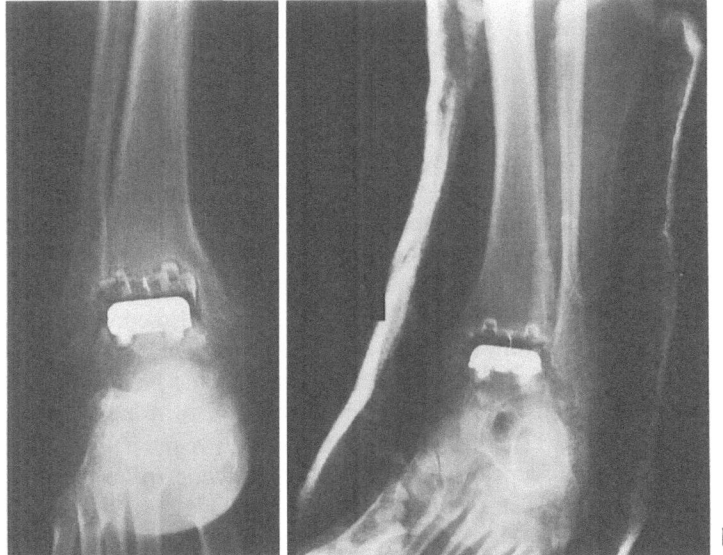

Fig. 6 a,b. Anteroposterior roentgenograms of the patient in Fig. 5 after Mayo Total Ankle Replacement

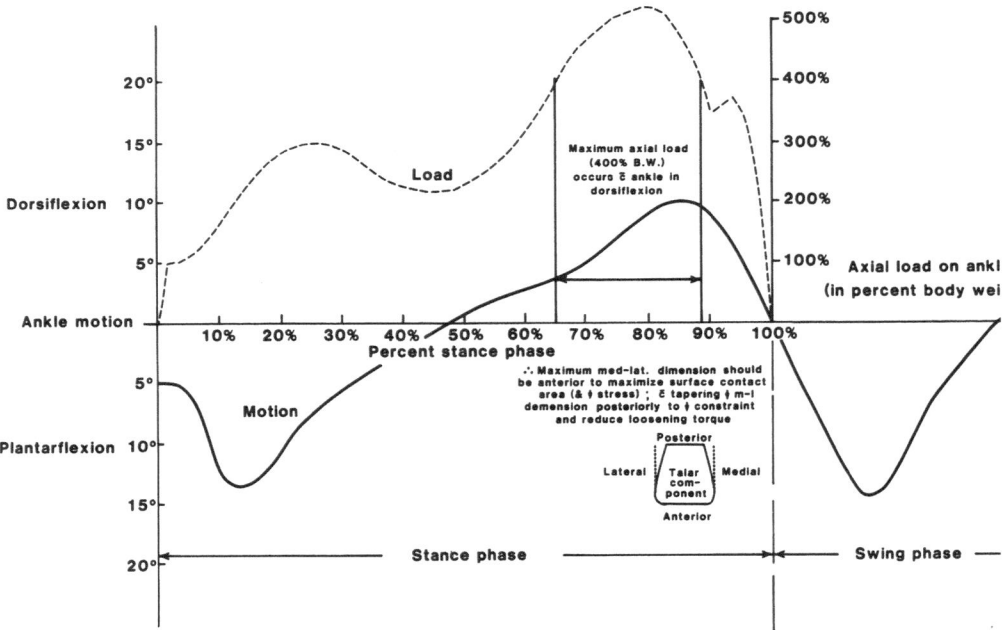

Fig. 7. Simultaneous plot of ankle joint motion and compressive load across the ankle during gait. The peak loads occur when the ankle is in dorsiflexion. Note that the maximum medio-lateral dimension should be anterior to maximize surface contact area, and lower stress, with tapering lowering the m-l dimension posteriorly to lower constraint and reduce loosening torque

Considering the designs of TAR used in the United States and Europe, the Mayo design is categorized as cylindrical and totally congruent — providing uniplanar stable motion. Studies of torsional resistance show the Mayo TAR to be equally as strong as a normal ankle, reducing the likelihood for impact failure of the bone or ligament attachments. On the other hand, this means that torsional loading trans-mits torque to the bone (cement) prosthesis interfaces and may account for the loosening seen. The spherical design of TAR is also congruent but allows motion in all 3 planes like a universal joint. Its stability is poor, but the torque transmitted into the bone is less, therefore the loosening rate should be less. However, this has not yet been demonstrated in clinical studies. It would seem that the ideal TAR design lies somewhere between these two extremes, i.e., a partially constrained design. The design criteria of a prosthesis with only partial constraint means a mismatch in radii of curvature between the articulating parts. This results in reduced surface contact area and high contact stress; thus, deformation and excessive wear would be expected.

Since maximum loading occurs between 65% and 90% of the stance phase of gait — with the ankle in dorsiflexion (Fig. 7), it seems optional to ensure the maximum surface contact areas at this range. Thus, our new concept is to maintain the same radii of curvature, but to make the talar component wider in front so that the contact

Fig. 8. Prototype modification of total ankle prosthesis. Note the wider anterior dimension of the talar component which increases surface contact area and the narrower posterior dimension which allows less constraint, more rotation, and possibly less torque transmitted to the prosthesis/bone interface

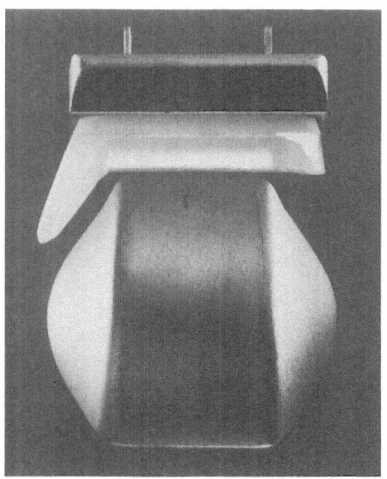

area is greater in dorsiflexion (where maximal loading occurs) and less in plantar flexion. This also would allow the ankle to rotate somewhat in plantar flexion. It so happens that this is the normal anatomic configuration of the talus. Figure 8 shows the current design. The polyethylene tibial component is encased in metal to reduce deformation and shear stress at the adjacent bone cement interface. The new device has anchoring fins on both components and the outer surfaces are coated with vitallium beads to allow bony ingrowth, and possible cementless fixation.

Although the results of total ankle replacement have been disappointing overall, results in the elderly OA and RA patients have been satisfactory. Achievement of better results in the younger, more active patient should be attainable with further study and refinement of prosthetic design parameters.

References

1. Fjermeros H, Hagen, R (1967) Posttraumatic arthrosis in the ankle and foot treated with arthrodesis. Acta Chir Scand 133:527
2. Johnson EW Jr, Boseker EH (1968) Arthrodesis of the ankle. Arch Surg 97:766
3. Lance EM, Pavel A, Patterson RL, Jr, Fries I, Larson IJ (1971) Arthrodesis of the ankle: A follow-up study. J Bone Joint Surg 53:A1030
4. Morrey BF, Weideman GP Jr (1980) Complications and long-term results of ankle arthrodeses following trauma. J Bone Joint Surg 62:A777
5. Stauffer RN, Chao EYS, Brewster RC (1977) Force and motion analysis of the normal, diseased, and prosthetic ankle joint. Clin Orthop 127:189
6. Stauffer RN, Segal NM (1981) Total ankle arthroplasty: Four years' experience. Clin Orthop 160:217
7. Stauffer RN (1982) Salvage of painful total ankle arthroplasty. Clin Orthop 170:184

Discussion III

Kawai (Kobe University): We have heard extensively about the biomecchanics of the foot and ankle. The force at the ankle is as much as five-fold body weight and the motion needed for function. When an implant is used there is a high rate of radiolucency and loosening thus the need for research to solve the problems of total ankle replacement (TAR).

Fujii (Himeji St. Maria Hospital): I am very interested in the function of the subtalar joint. We have heard that the hinged motion at the subtalar joint and there is rotational gliding in the varus and valgus. How does this occur?

Stauffer (Mayo Clinic): Gliding in the anterior/posterior plane occurs in dorsi and plantar flexion of the ankle joint, and to a much lesser extent at the subtalar joint. In patients with an ankle joint fusion, a greater degree of movement occurs in the subtalar joint up to double the usual motion there.

Kawai: On the topic of joint surgery, let us now discuss the design of the artificial joint. There are three main types of designs but ankle motion includes hinged motion together with rotational gliding. What is the optimal design for the semi-constrained or non-constrained TAR?

Onishi (Osaka National Hospital): I have experience with 10 TAR in rheumatoid arthritis (RA) cases. Motion has been poor but pain relief good. We did see radiolucency at the implant/bone interface. At the tibia, we saw lucent zones in cases with poor bone but when these weak areas were packed the lucency was less.

On the tibial side, the polyethylene is very thin which may predispose creep deformation. Does creep occur if there is a metal back on the prosthesis? We use ceramics, some with and some without cement. On the tibial side, radiolucency is more common in those without cement. I think this is due to the small contact areas and the high load per square centimeter of the artifical joint.

Tateishi (Hyogo Medical University): When the talus is severely damaged, I believe anchorage using cement down to the calcaneus is dangerous. What is your opinion, Dr. Stauffer?

Stauffer: I agree. One must have adequate viable living bone to anchor the device. One must not violate the subtalar joint by cement or a fin of the talar component, as it will lead to destructive lesions and pain. When there is insufficient bone, the patient is not a good candidate for TAR of any design.

Yoshino (Tokyo): Dr. Stauffer, regarding the tibial component and the technique for its insertion, I believe it is very difficult. From my experience, the tibial component is often malplaced, angulated posteriorly. Would a cutting jig prevent this?

Stauffer: You are quite right that the positioning of ankle devices is difficult. We must develop instrumentation to allow us to place the prosthetic device properly from front to back. If it is located too far anteriorly, the axis of rotation is also too far forward — then the device simply gaps open. We are developing better instrumentation with the new device.

Yoshino: If the talo-calcaneal joint is arthritic and painful, what measures do you recommend?

Stauffer: We don't have a good answer to that either. If osteophytes impinge we excise them. In the consideration of all of the TAR devices available, like the early history of THR and TKR, at the present time none of the devices used for TAR are ideal, but should evolve over time. This delay in development has a number of reasons. Few are interested in this problem and industry is not interested in putting money or effort into development because it is a low volume sales item. This is sad because there are a number of people in the world who have bad ankle problems for whom ankle fusion is not optimal.

Onishi: In revision cases, did you assess the polyethylene surfaces? Did creep occur?

Stauffer: The answer is yes. Creep deformation of the tibial component was present in all of the revised cases. The medial and lateral lips were deformed and the surface flattened, which means that the talar component is attempting to rotate inside the tibial component. Design of a semi-constrained form which is metal backed should permit some rotation and lessen contact stresses and any loosening tendancy.

Kawai: Dr. Mann and Dr. Stauffer, both of you have many years of experience in this field. I have three questions for you. (1) What is the best indication? (2) What is the optimal current design? (3) Should cement be used?

Stauffer: Ankle fusion is our best choice in the majority of cases. But in RA and elderly OA cases, where physical demands are limited, then TAR is reasonable.

Mann (University of California): I basically agree, but one needs to consider several other factors. In post-traumatic ankle arthritis, although the trauma may appear primarily in the ankle joint, often the subtalar joint has also sustained significant damage. This is one of the reasons why successful TAR may have persisting disability, such as stiffness or arthritis of the subtalar joint. Isolated disease in the older patient or in the rheumatoid, is a reasonable case for TAR. My preference is still an ankle arthrodesis. I have done many and had success. I do not consider the morbidity from ankle fusion to be so major even in a person with severe RA with multiple joint involvement.

Although TAR is a useful tool in our armamentarian, probably one of the reasons why it has not developed further is because we already have a good operation (fusion) and the loss of ankle joint motion is nowhere nearly as severe a problem as loss of hip and knee joint motion.

Stauffer: But you have already indicated that the stresses on the subtalar joint are markedly magnified after ankle arthrodesis. Do you believe that you are not doing any damage by fusing an ankle joint and imposing an increased stress on an already diseased subtalar and midtarsal joint in rheumatoids arthritic patients? Also, what about added stresses to the contra-lateral knee?

Mann: I think that in rheumatoids most are not walking normally and the force involved is probably anywhere from 30–50 percent less than usual. That is why they tolerate these problems better than normals.

Kawai: We certainly expect that there will be more research and consequently better prospects for TAR in the future.

Part 2
Problem Case Presentation and
Surgical Decision Making

Segmental Comminuted Open Supracondylar Fracture of the Distal Femur

KOSAKU MIZUNO[1]

Introduction

This is a case report of a 37-year-old housewife who was involved in a traffic accident on November 9, 1986, sustaining major trauma to the right leg. She was brought to the emergency room of a hospital within an hour. According to the orthopaedic surgeon in charge of her initial care, the injury was diagnosed as a Type III [1] open contaminated fracture of the femur communicating with the knee joint. Nerve and distal vascular supply were intact. The 10 cm × 1.5 cm transverse wound crossing the suprapatellar area contained glass fragments and pieces of clothing.

Radiographic Findings

The radiographs revealed a segmental comminuted supracondylar T fracture with many foreign body densities representing the glass fragments. The patella was displaced inferiorly (Fig. 1).

Question and Answer 1

Which Primary Treatment Is Best?

Okada (Rokko Hospital): I would remove everything that could lead to infection and use an external fixator from the center of the femur to the middle tibia. A plaster may be used as an alternative.

Chandler (Harvard Medical School): If the major nerves were distally damaged with an insensate distal extremity, I would consider primary amputation. Otherwise, I would proceed to massive debridement followed initially by tibial pin traction.

[1] Department of Orthopedic Surgery, Kobe University School of Medicine, Kobe, Japan

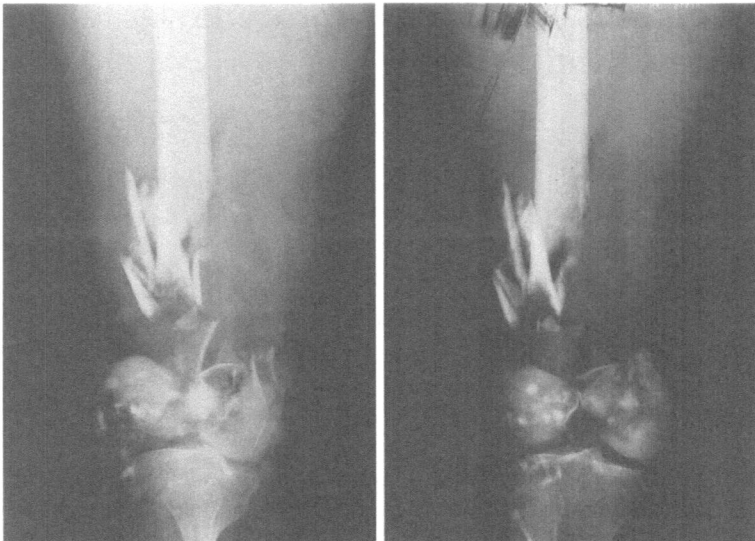

Fig. 1. At time of injury

Stauffer (Mayo Clinic): One other initial consideration is to resect the patella and reconstruct the patellar tendon mechanism. I think it is important to do that early. If you wait to reconstruct the quadriceps and patella mechanism, you cannot expect a good outcome.

Wilde (Cleveland Clinic): The only added comment is to maintain leg length. I would use an external fixator. It also enhances patient care.

Initial Treatment: Initial treatment included wide debridement, removing numerous glass fragments, pieces of clothing and small devitalized bone fragments. Damaged soft tissues were excised and the wounds were cleansed with large volumes of saline. The wounds were closed primarily and a long leg splint was applied. The patient was transferred to our university hospital 7 days after injury.

Late Wound Therapy

When assessed, the wound appeared clean but there was some discharge from the suture line and some local heat and swelling. As shown in Table 1, the laboratory analyses of erythrocyte sedimentation rate (ESR), C-reactive protein (CRP) and white blood cell count (WBC) worsened (Table 1). However, no organism was found in wound aspirates and the patient remained afebrile.

Radiographs still revealed some pieces of glass with the bone defects among the fractured fragments (Fig. 2). The wound was carefully observed, with the leg in a long cast, and intravenous and oral antibiotics were administered (Cephalosporin, 2 g per day for 4 weeks).

Table 1. Results of blood analyses

Date of test	ESR (mm/1 per hour)	WBC	CRP (mg/l)	Culture
November 18, 1986[a]	88	7900	33	negative
November 20, 1986	98	9100	33	negative

ESR, erythrocyte sedimentation rate; WBC, white blood cell count; CRP, C-reactive protein
[a] Admission to hospital

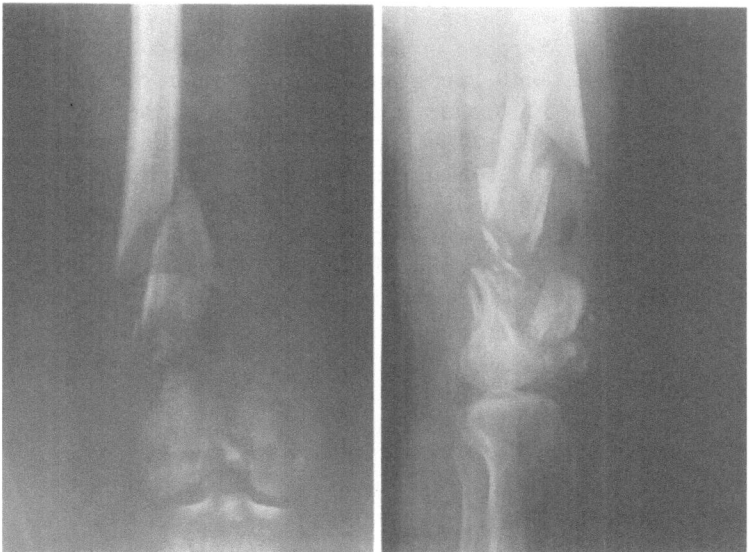

Fig. 2. After initial debridement

Question and Answer 2

What Should Be Done at This Time?

Ohno (Sanda): I would delay surgery, using external fixation to preserve the leg length and stability.

Ohnishi (Osaka): I agree.

Stauffer: I would not use primary closure because this was a massively contaminated injury. I would perform initial debridement and leave the wound open with delayed closure at 48h with secondary debridement prior to closure. More precisely, I would debride the wound extensively and repair the quadriceps mechanism, remove the patella, and secure the fracture with an external fixator. I would probably not close the wound at this stage but debride it after 48h before final closure.

Chandler: I agree with the secondary debridement, but I would close the wound to cover the knee joint with an anterior fixator.

Huang (Beijing): I would use a joint brace or external fixation. I would wait for the second stage to do another operation when the glass may be removed.

Treatment: A second debridement was performed, removing blood clots, many glass fragments and more bits of the clothing she was wearing. However, there was no pus. Massive irrigation was then performed. The wound was closed and continuous irrigation was set up. Wagner's apparatus was applied to correct the alignment and for splinting the leg. Continuous irrigation was maintained for 2 weeks with definite improvement. The ESR returned to the normal level, the WBC was approximately 5,600, and CRP decreased to below 0.2 mg/dl. The healing of the wound was clean.

At surgery the torn quadriceps mechanism was repaired, but the patella was not removed. The knee joint surfaces were well preserved with a few anterior and inter-condylar fracture lines. The external fixator was applied with two pins inserted into the central part of the femur proximally and two more pins inserted into the tibia beyond the knee joint. No further special treatment was performed for 3 months.

Treatment of the Bone Defect

The condition of the distal thigh, including the skin, was quite good. A large bone defect was evident on the X-ray (Fig. 3). Biochemical examination showed no particular abnormality.

Question and Answer 3

How Should the 12-cm Bone Loss Be Managed?

Chandler: I would fasten the two condyles with multiple screws, then connect that segment to the proximal one with an AO plate and fill the intervening gap with bone graft or an allograft with supplementary bone graft.

Mann (University of California): Can knee motion ever be re-established again? At 3 months, the probability approaches zero. Thus, to obtain bone union with rigid fixation is a priority, and then a cast brace should be used to mobilize the knee. I would use a blade plate or a clover leaf plate with an iliac bone graft.

Stauffer: It is going to be very difficult at 3 months; perhaps optimally, surgery at 2 weeks to fix the condyles and then wait to deal with the diaphyseal fracture. I would use a right-angle compression screw and plate. A vascularized fibular graft might be considered. I would not likely deal with the functional knee.

Fig. 3. At 3 months after the second debridement and external fixation

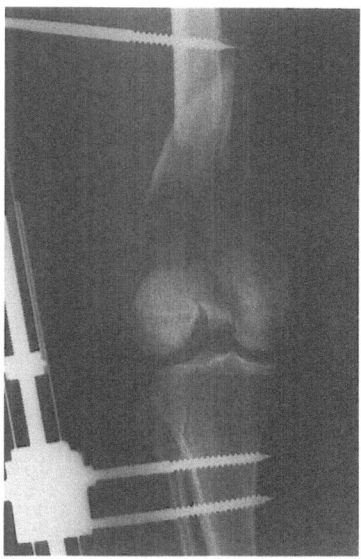

Wilde: I would not use continuous irrigation due to the risks of secondary infection. At the second debridement, I would have fixed the large free fragment of the femur with AO fragmentary screws and lessened the bone defect. The condyles of the femur may also be fixed, and then wait for the wound to declare itself. I would choose to use an AO blade plate and a bone graft with allograft.

Cooke: At this stage the wound might have been approached with the Papineau technique, using a cancellous bone graft to the defect and a supracondylar plate. If necessary, I would leave it open if there is any question about sepsis.

Bone Grafting

Bone grafting of both fibular and iliac bones was performed and the external fixation was left intact. As shown on the post-operative X-ray (Fig. 4), the bone grafting does not seem to be sufficient, as there is a gap on the medial side. There were some technical limitations due to dense fibrous tissues.

After bone grafting, the fixation was maintained for 4 months without weight bearing. After removal of the external fixator, a long leg brace with partial weight bearing was used for 3 months. The new bone then started to grow into the defect with remarkable remodelling, sufficient to tolerate full weight bearing. One year after the injury, the patient could walk without support (Fig. 5). Her knee motion however, is only 0° to 30°. She has no specific complaint of pain, only the limitation of knee motion. She has little active extension due to adhesion of the distal quadriceps, including the patella and its tendon. We have been reluctant to attempt to surgically mobilize her stiff knee as that may cause more damage and pain.

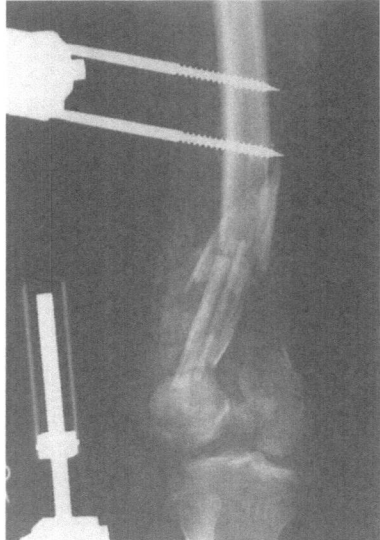

Fig. 4. After bone grafting

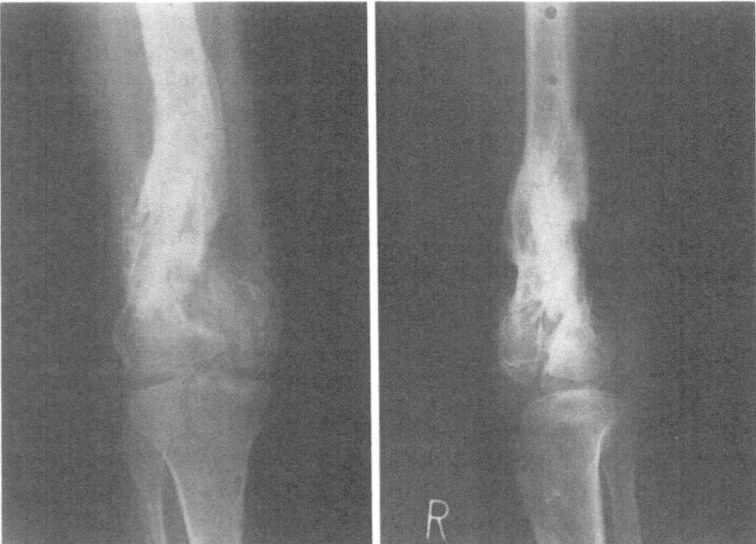

Fig. 5. At 1 year after injury

Discussion

Major open comminuted fractures of the knee are difficult treatment problems.
Four management points must be considered: debridement, fixation of the fractured
bone, bone loss, and reconstruction of the knee joint.

In the present case, initial debridement at the emergency hospital was inadequate and primary wound closure was inadvisable [2]. The two most important steps are to make the contaminated wound a clean wound to promote rapid healing of the soft tissue and to clean and close the potentially infected fracture [2-4]. In this case, continuing signs of inflammation clearly necessitated a second debridement and at that time devitalized soft tissue, debris, and bone were completely excised. Regarding fracture fixation, here a splint would hamper patient care, however an external fixator would enhance it. Treatment of the fractured bone is as a rule, a secondary step but it may be of value to enhance soft tissue healing. The disadvantages of internal fixation, such as use of a blade plate, are the added damage to the soft tissue during application and increase in soft tissue tension [5]. Wound infection could complicate the problem with osteomyelitis [6].

In bone grafting, a longer delay may lessen the possibility of infection [1]. Here, a month may have been sufficient and may have also enhanced joint motion. The source of bone for the graft is autogenous at best; cancellous is the most effective. Fibrous tissue in-between the fractured fragments has the potential for new bone formation, thus here it was unnecessary to perform a further graft for a vascularized graft [6]. Regarding the reconstruction of the stiff knee, it was unnecessary to reconstruct the knee joint as the extension mechanism had been damaged.

Conclusion

A severely comminuted open fracture of the distal femur was presented for discussion of the treatment procedure. Radical debridement was immediately necessary, prior to any other treatment. Secondary iliac bone graft with external fixation proved beneficial for the bone defect at the fractured site. It is recommended to proceed with the reconstruction of a stiff knee, as a lengthy delay may hamper knee mobility.

References

1. Gustilo RB, et al (1976) Prevention of infection in the treatment of 1,025 open fractures of long bones: Retrospective and prospective analysis. J Bone Joint Surg 58A: 453
2. Patzakis MJ, et al (1975) The early management of open joint injuries: a prospective study of 140 patients. J Bone Joint Surg 57A: 1065
3. Barfred T, et al (1973) Myoplasty for covering exposed bone or joint on the lower leg. Acta Orthop Scand 44: 532
4. Benson DR, et al (1983) Treatment of open fractures: a prospective study. J Trauma 23: 25
5. Anderson JT, et al (1980) Immediate internal fixation in open fractures. Orthop Clin North Am 11: 569
6. Copeland CX Jr, et al (1965) Incidence of osteomyelitis in compound fractures. Am J Surg 31: 156

Management of Splayfoot: Report of a Case

Masahiro Kurosaka, Hirotsugu Muratsu, and Kosaku Mizuno[1]

Our case is a 15-year-old high school girl. At the age of 8 years, she first noticed a splayfoot deformity, which, began causing pain at the 5th metatarsophalangeal (MTP) joint at the age 12. Since then, she has had difficulty finding comfortable shoes. The symptoms became worse and the only shoes she could wear other than sneakers were lace-up shoes (Fig. 1). When she was seen at our hospital, marked splayfoot deformity was found bilaterally. Although weight-bearing accentuated the deformity, there was no hallux valgus or flatfoot deformity noted. A tailor's bunion had formed on the lateral side of each 5th MTP joint which was very tender (Fig. 2). On weight-bearing roentgenogram, the 1st and 2nd intermetatarsal angles appeared within the normal range (12° on the right foot and 10° on the left). The obvious abnormalities noticed were the increased intermetatarsal angles between the 4th and 5th metatarsals and the 1st and 5th (Fig. 3). Both angles were increased on weight-bearing. In the lateral view, the medial longitudinal arch was maintained (Fig. 4).

Fig. 1. The pair of lace-up shoes which the patient used on her visit to the clinic

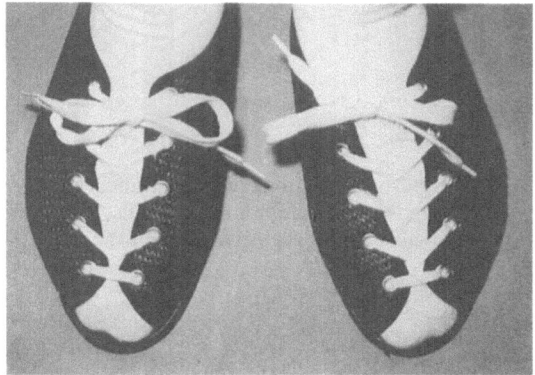

[1] Department of Orthopedic Surgery, Kobe University School of Medicine, Kobe, Japan

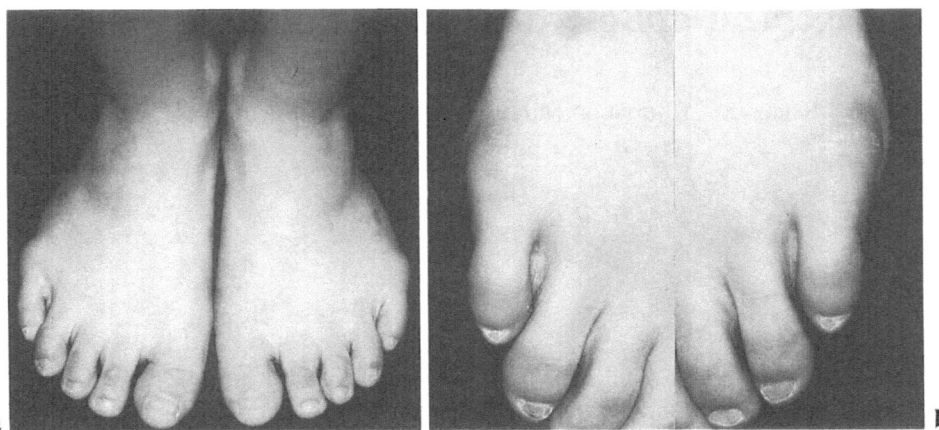

Fig. 2 a Although splayfoot deformity is marked, no hallux valgus deformity is noted in this clinical photograph of both feet. **b** Lateral sides of both 5th metatarsophalangeal (MTP) joints. Note the tender tailor's bunions

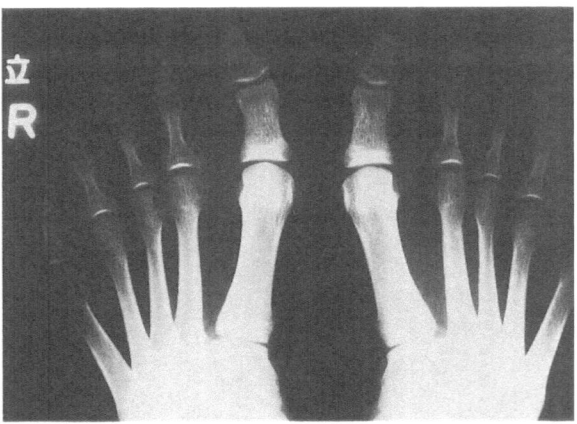

Fig. 3. Weight-bearing dorsoplantar radiograph demonstrates increased intermetatarsal angles between the 4th and 5th metatarsals (16° on the *right*, 15° on the *left*) and the 1st and 5th metatarsals (40° on the *right*, 38° on the *left*)

Question and Answers 1

What Type of Conservative Treatment Should Be Given?

Chairman, *Mizuno* (Kobe University): May we have some ideas from the floor? Dr. Fujii, what is your opinion?

Fig. 4. Weight-bearing lateral
radiograph demonstrated no
flatfoot deformity

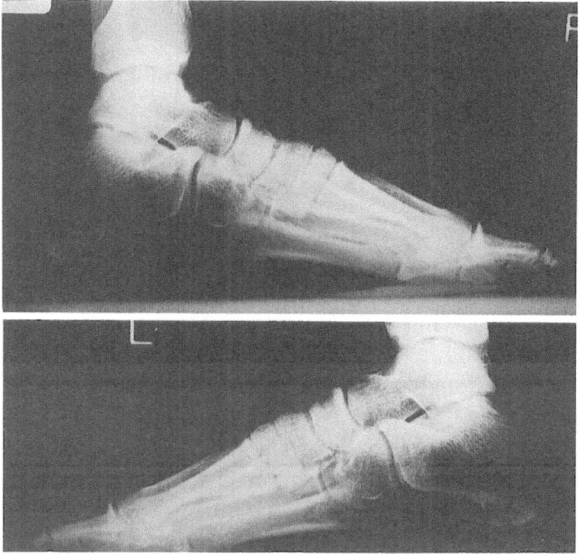

Fujii (Himeji St. Maria Hospital): Strengthening the muscles, especially plantar muscle exercises would be of benefit to a certain extent. Also, a metatarsal pad to support the transverse arch might be useful.

Chairman: Dr. Mann, any comments on conservative management?

Mann (University of California): Before talking about conservative management, I would like to ask you two questions. First, does she have generalized hyperlaxity? Second, does she have a lesion underneath the 5th metatarsal head, or is the entire problem the lesion laterally over the 5th metatarsal head?

Kurosaka: She does not have generalized laxity nor has a lesion underneath the metatarsal head.

Mann: I think, as far as conservative treatment is concerned, only a wide shoe is indicated. At the same time, you must be sure that there are no seams in the shoe over the area where the pain is coming from. I do not think an insert will help this patient very much. The more you add to her shoe, the more pressure over the involved area she will have.

As Dr. Mann suggested, her pain was not alleviated by the use of a shoe insert. Although the transverse arch was restored with the insert, she had difficulty getting her feet into the shoes. As she continued to experience pain, we considered the necessity of surgical treatment.

Question and Answer 2

What Type of Surgical Treatment Would Be Helpful?

Chairman: Although we very rarely see splayfoot in Japan, do you have any comments on the surgical treatment, Dr. Fujii?

Fujii: My experience in surgical treatment of this problem is limited to two cases. I would recommend open-wedge osteotomy at the base of the 1st and 5th metatarsals.

Chairman: What is your opinion, Dr. Mann?

Mann: Athough we do not operate for splayfoot very often, in a case such as this, I would suggest a long, oblique, midshaft 5th-metatarsal osteotomy [1]. The distal portion of the metatarsus should be shifted medialward, and the osteotomy site should be fixed with a 3.5 mm AO screw. I prefer midshaft, because the incidence of nonunion is higher if you go too far towards the base. In a situation where there is no lateral deviation of the 5th metatarsal shaft, an osteotomy of the lateral aspect of the metatarsl head is sufficient. However, in this case you need to do a midshaft osteotomy.

Operative Management

Modified Giannestras osteotomy was conducted [2, 3]. Open wedge osteotomy was performed on the bases of the 1st and 5th metatarsals, and the heads of the 1st and 5th metatrsals were transfixed with threaded pins while the 1st and 5th intermetatarsal angles were held corrected. Tailor's bunions over the 5th MTP joint and the bony projection of the 5th metatarsal head were trimmed. At the same time, the 1st and 2nd intermetatarsal ligaments and the 4th and 5th intermetatarsal ligaments were tightened to maintain the correction. The immediate postoperative radiograph showed good correction of the 1st and 5th intermetatarsal angles ($20°$ on the right foot and $16°$ on the left) (Fig. 5). She was placed in short-leg casts for 6 weeks. One year later, the radiographs showed that the correction of the 1st and 5th intermetatarsal angle was well maintained ($21°$ on the right foot and $17°$ on the left) (Fig. 6). At the time of writing, she was able to run without pain and wear off-the-shelf shoes without major difficulties.

Discussion

Generally, splayfoot deformity is reported most often in patients with rheumatoid arthritis or generalized connective tissue abnormalities such as Ehlers-Danlos syndrome. Also, in most of these cases, splayfoot is combined with flatfoot and or hallux valgus deformity. In this respect, our case, a 15-year-old girl without any underlying disease or other abnormality, was somewhat unusual. As to the management of splayfoot, conservative means such as selection of wider shoes and plantar

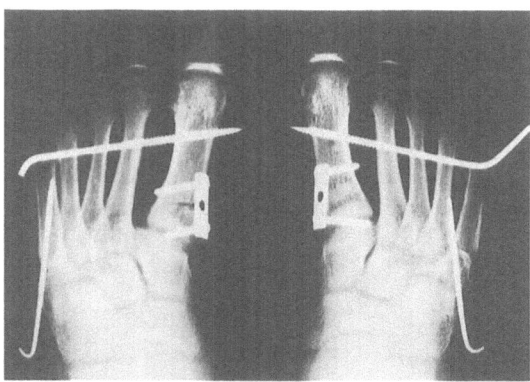

Fig. 5. Postoperative radiograph with correction of splayfoot deformity. The 1st and 5th inter-metatarsal angle is 20° on the *right* and 16° on the *left*

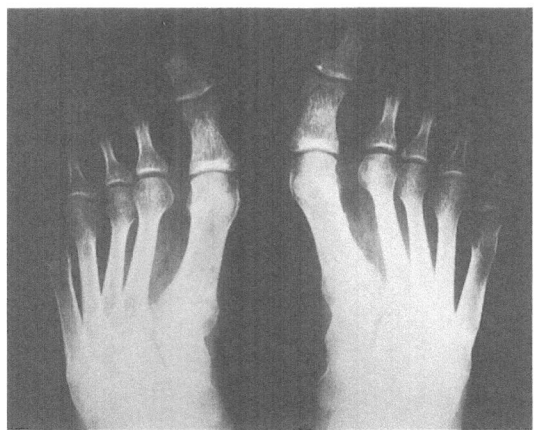

Fig. 6. Postoperative radiograph taken at the 1-year follow-up visit

muscle exercise are often beneficial in many cases. Although our patient sought any shoes available, pain on the lateral aspect of the 5th MTP joint was a tenacious complaint and led us to operative treatment.

Concerning surgical procedures, correction of splayfoot can be achieved by either osteotomy or soft-tissue procedures. The most popular soft-tissue surgery is the Jopling procedure [3], which is also known as the soft-tissue sling procedure. In this procedure, the long extensor tendon of the 5th digit, transected at the level of the ankle joint, is used as a sling to tie together the spread metatarsal heads. Although few complications were reported by Jopling, we believe splayfoot is a structural abnormality, which should be corrected by bone realignment. Osseous procedures such as the Giannestras procedure will allow for more predictable correction, because recurrence caused by stretching of ligamentous and tendinous structures is eliminated.

Although we performed open-wedge osteotomy on the base of the metatarsus, oblique osteotomy at midshaft is one alternative for the correction of this problem. Use of either technique, properly performed on appropriately chosen patients, offers surgical correction of splayfoot deformity with a predictable end result.

References

1. Yu GV, Ruch JA, Smith TF (1987) Deformity and surgery of the fifth ray. In: McGlamry (ed) Comprehensive textbook of foot surgery. Vol. I. Williams and Wilkins, Baltimore, pp 114–132
2. Bishop J, Kahn A, Turba JE (1980) Surgical Correction of the splayfoot: The Giannestras procedure. Clin Orthop 146: 234–235
3. Cowell HR (1983) Splay foot. In: Evarts CM (ed) Surgery of the musculokeletal system. Vol. 4. Churchill and Livingstone, New York, pp 9: 173–180

Application of Machining Principles: Use of the Questor Saw Jig in TKR for Severe Valgus Hyperextension Osteoarthritis of the Knee

T. Derek V. Cooke[1]

This case report concerns a 65-year-old female with severe bilateral knee OA and the application of machining technology in her treatment with a total knee replacement (TKR). Ten years before, this patient had had bilateral patellectomies. On the right this was complicated by an iatrogenic rupture of the quadriceps mechanism such that she could not actively extend the knee. She developed increasingly severe pain due to OA which was much greater on the left. The right knee was in varus and only stable when standing in extension. She could get around only with a walker and this caused terrible pain in the lateral compartment of the left knee. Standardized radiographs confirmed severe valgus and hyperextension of the left knee with collapse of the lateral compartment; a widely gaping medial compartment and some anterior subluxation of the tibia was also noted (Fig. 1a, b).

We decided to operate on the left knee because it was so painful and would not support her in rehabilitation of right knee surgery. Under anesthesia she had very marked valgus deformity with wide medial opening (Fig. 2); with varus stress we could not quite correct the valgus. The hyperextension was associated with anterior translation of the tibia.

Question and Answer

How Do We Go about Correction of This Problem?

Tateishi (Hyogo Medical University): I would opt for TKR. The iliotibial band laterally needs to be transversely released with the lateral retinaculum. The medial side needs to be tightened.

Chairman, *Mizuno* (Kobe University): So soft tissue release of the knee is advised with TKR. Is there another view?

Inoue (Okayama University): I agree with Dr. Tateishi. We need to adjust the extensor mechanism and balance the soft tissue intraoperatively. But in surgery, I think it is very important to tighten the medial collateral ligament (MCL) and other soft tissues so that there will be some flexion.

[1] Clinical Mechanics Group, Queen's University, Kingston, Ontario, Canada

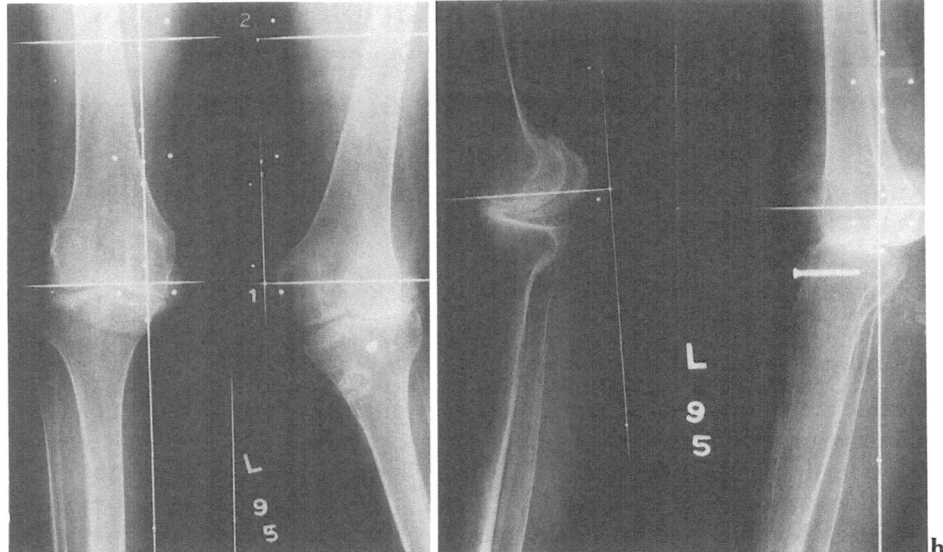

Fig. 1 a,b. Pre-operative standardized radiographs of both knees. Note severe valgus hyperextension on the left and widely gaping medial compartment

Chairman: Are there any further views? Dr. Ohno, are you of the same opinion?

Ohno (Sanda Hospital): To what extent was the extensor mechanism preserved? nism preserved?

Cooke (Queen's University): It was working fine on the left side even without a patella.

Ohno: In that case, I agree with the opinions expressed.

Chairman: So we have a consensus from the Japanese doctors. What about the overseas group?

Wilde (Cleveland Clinic): I would prefer to release the tight ligaments on the lateral side and use a posteriorly stabilized condyler TKR prosthesis with cement.

Stauffer (Mayo Clinic): I would agree with the lateral release. I do not know what the timing was in the development of this deformity, but I would be very worried about the recurrence of valgus deformity in that knee, because she is getting out of a chair with a stiff knee on the right side. If one watches a rheumatoid patient or anyone with a stiff knee getting out of a chair, the opposite knee goes into tremendous valgus. Thus if we just brace the right knee, even though we have a very nicely balanced TKR, the valgus deformity might recur. So while I would agree with Dr. Wilde, I think we also need to think very seriously about doing something about the quadriceps mechanism on the right side as well.

Fig. 2. Under anesthesis the knee showed
severe medial laxity

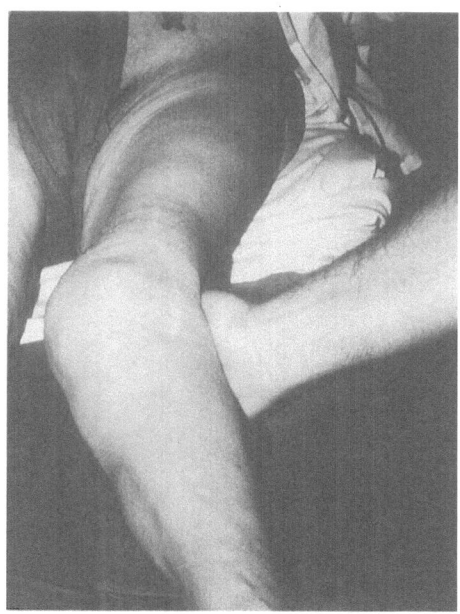

Chandler (Harvard Medical School): I basically agree that we should do TKR on the
left side with a lot of release. I would not hesitate to tighten the medial side. There
was some discussion today about the posterior cruciate ligament (PCL), which I per-
sonally feel is very important to leave. I think that the quadriceps and the PCL are
synergistic. I would not take the PCL but use an unconstrained prosthesis, probably
a cemented PCL conserving TKR, with lateral release.

Operative Management

The degree of hyperflexibility in this patient was also a big concern. At surgery we
approached the joint anterolaterally elevating the tibial tubercle. This approach
gives excellent access to tight lateral structures. The operative findings showed gross
loss of cartilage with a deep excavation of the lateral tibia, marked chondrocal-
cinosis, and no anterior cruciate ligament (ACL), but a well-preserved PCL. The iliotibial band and lateral retinaculum were released as well as the lateral capsule and
popliteous tendon. This corrected the valgus deformity.

The knee was then set up in the Questor Saw Jig (Fig. 3a). The distractor hook
was located at the origin of the PCL [1]. The tibia was aligned with the long axis
parallel to the distal frame, neutrally rotated, and then held with a transfixation pin
(Fig. 3b). The knee was distracted at 90° flexion, the frame and tibia were aligned to
the hip, as confirmed by anterior-posterior (AP) X-ray, and the femur was rotated to
neutral. The transepicondylar plane was parallel to the transverse apical bar of the
frame and then the femur was transfixed (see pp. 59–65)

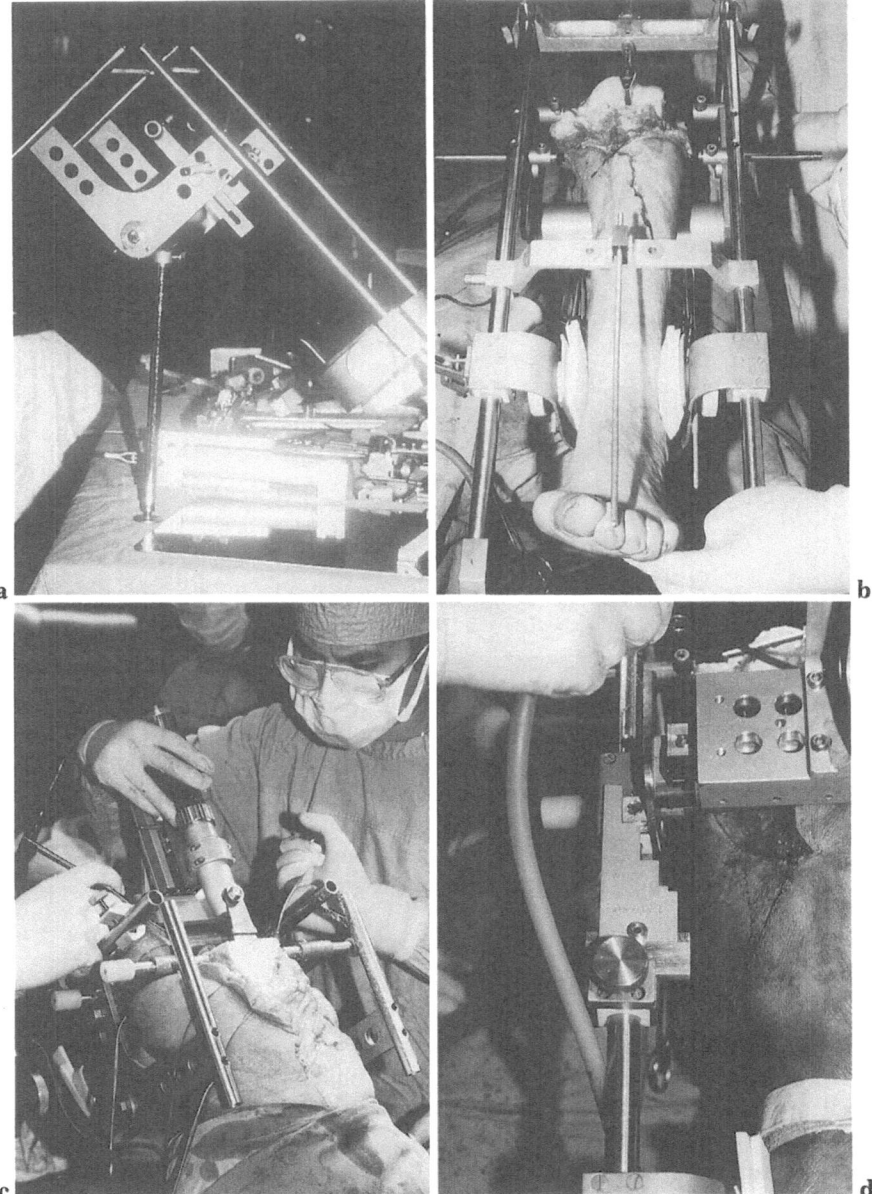

Fig. 3 a-d. Operative view of the Questor Saw Jig in use for total knee replacement in this case. **a** Saw bench 90° frame. **b** Frontal view of knee held proximally by the distractor hook at the posterior cruciate ligament attachment, distally aligned with the frame. Fixation was made by a transfixing proximal tibial pin. **c** Triaxial saw mounted on the proximal arms of the frame. Precise bone cuts are made without excessive debris. **d** Template used for Townley medium prosthesis. *O*, reference for posterior cruciate ligament; *1*, anterior femoral cut; *2*, posterior femoral cut; *3* tibial proximal cut

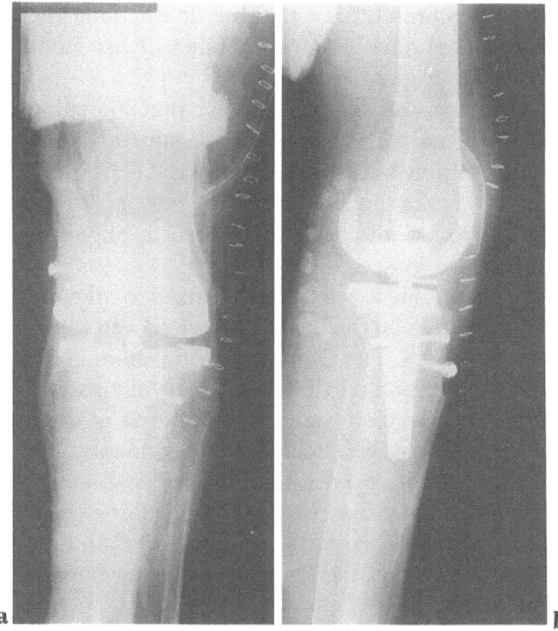

Fig. 4 a,b. Post-operative radiograph showing implant positioning well aligned to hip and ankle with correction of deformity

Once the knee was aligned on each bone's axis, at 90° flexion and fixed, the distractor was removed and the triaxial saw mounted (Fig. 3c). Femoral end bearing and proximal tibial cuts were each made precisely, according to the interior dimensions of the Townley prosthesis using a pre-determined template (Fig. 3d), size matched as the best fit to the bone. The defeat in the lateral tibial plateau was bone grafted and the bone gap remaining made up by an extra thick tibial component plastic insert. Thus we resected minimal bone, preserved the PCL, made up bone with graft, made bone cuts aligned to the hip and ankle, orienting each prosthetic component to neutral (on the respective mechanical axis) and maintained the joint line level (at 90° to load-bearing axis). With the trials in place the re-alignment was excellent, the hyperextension gone, but the medial collateral ligament (MCL) was still slack. The origin was therefore approximated to take up the slack. Thus the PCL, capsule and medial soft tissues were put in tension. Implants were inserted, the tibia being cemented (Fig. 4a, b).

Discussion

While it is easier to obtain a correct alignment by resecting the cruciate ligaments you then need to use a more restrained prosthetic design, such as the posterior stabilized knee, to maintain stability; the joint line then becomes elevated. However, if the PCL is present then making up the bone gap with a thicker tibial plateau on top of preserved remaining good bone will also stabilize the knee and maintain the joint line at its original level.

The now well established fact that loosening of TKR and impaired kinemetics relate to malposition and malalignment (see pp. 59–65) stimulated our group to develop a precise technology for TKR [1]. This technique embodies machining principles to make precise debris free saw cuts of each bone referenced accurately to the hip and ankle with each bone correctly aligned and held in a frame, on its respective mechanical axis.

In machining a work bench is used to align and hold the work piece and a cutting tool, mounted on the bench, is then moved to the appropriate location in order to cut the work piece. The Questor Saw Jig embodies these ideas: A frame at 90° is used to hold the femur and tibia each neutrally rotated and aligned parallel to the frame limbs. A distractor attached to the apex of the frame and applied to a central kinematic point the PCL, tensions the ligaments. The cutting tool used is a triaxial rotatable air (or battery) driven oscilating saw — other tools may be substituted. Dimensional cuts are defined by prefabricated templates accurately fashioned to replicate the interior prosthetic measurements of any desired knee. The saw is moved from point to point on the frame to cut each bone part accurately as referenced by the template.

Manufacturing precision of TKR implants of + / − 0.5 mm requires an equally precise tooling method for their accurate insertion. The Questor Saw Jig aims to duplicate this need by using principles applied in the manufacturing industry. Successful outcome of TKR should follow the application of these principles, lessening independent of specific instruments required by most current prostheses, provides a truly universal system by which different TKR designs may be compared.

Acknowledgments. The author wishes to acknowledge the valuable input of the Clinical Mechanics Group members in development of Questor Saw Jig.

Reference

1. Cooke TDV, Harada Y, Saunders G, Sliu D, Wevers H, Yoshioka YG (1988) Application of bench mounted saws for precision replacement arthroplasty of the arthritic knee — the Questor systems. In: Second Congress of the European Society (eds) Surgery and arthroscopy of the knee. Müller/Hackenbruch, Springer-Verlag, Berlin Heidelberg

Treatment of Infected Total Knee Arthroplasty

KAZUO KAWAI[1]

This case report concerns a 53-year-old female with infection of the left knee after total knee replacement (TKR) arthroplasty. She had a 15-year history of rheumatoid arthritis.

Two years earlier, this patient had had bilateral TKR and total hip replacement (THR) on the right. One and a half years after TKR, swelling on the medial side of the left knee became apparent (Fig. 1a), but no local heat or redness was found. The patient had slight pain on motion and tenderness around the medial mass. Ten ml of turbid, bloody fluid was aspirated from the medial swollen mass. Bacterial culture was negative. No apparent swelling was found in the knee joint. Our initial diagnosis was bursitis in the medial area of the knee. However, the X-ray showed osteolytic lesion in the medial side under the tibial component (Fig. 1b). Arthrography revealed a large, swollen bursa communicating with the tibial bone, which was identified as an osteolytic lesion (Fig. 1c). Moreover, *Staphylococcus epidermidis* was detected by repeated aspiration. Thus, it was definite that there was infection, probably in 2 localized area of the knee, but not in the entire joint. How was the treatment of this problem carried out?

Question and Answer

Chairman, *Cooke* (Queen's University): Dr. Wilde, in summary, the successful, new replacement in this rheumatoid patient is complicated now with septic bursitis and osteolytic lesion in the medial side of the tibia. But from what it looks like from the arthrogram and what appears in the localized area, what would you do?

Wilde (Cleveland Clinic): Well, I think the infection involves the knee joint, and we should remove the prosthesis and cement, and do a synovectomy. Certainly, I would get cultures from the bone-cement membrane and then put in a methacrylate spacer containing antibiotics. I would imagine that the therapy would be fairly sensitive. I do not know what your sensitivities are running here, but I would put antibiotic in the spacer. One of the antibiotics we are commonly using is tobramycin. The spacer has the effect of maintaining the length of the ligaments, and you do not

---

[1] Department of Orthopedic Surgery, Kobe University School of Medicine, Kobe, Japan

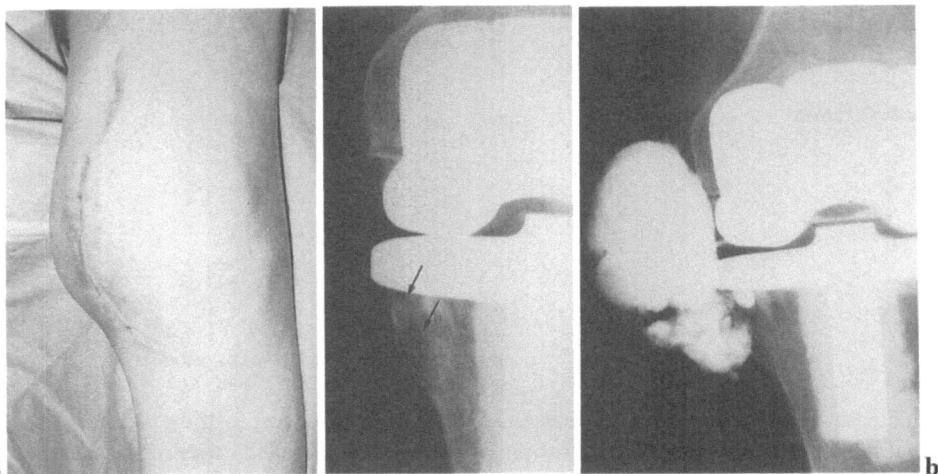

a   b,c

Fig. 1 a Apparent swelling on the medial side of the knee. Patient had total knee replacement 1½ years prior. **b** X-ray shows an osteolytic lesion on the medial side of the tibia under the prosthesis (*arrow*). **c** Arthrography revealed a large bursa and its communication to the bone where osteolysis was seen

need a plaster cast or any external fixation device. You would just mobilize with all that was necessary so that patient could get up afterwards, and then, with an aspirator on a weekly basis for 3 weeks. Now, if the first culture was sterile, then I would go back at 4 weeks, remove the spacer, debride it again, cutting a portion of the bone just a millimeter or 2 with a saw and reimplant a prosthesis with antibiotic and cement.

Chairman: Dr. Stauffer, any difference in opinion?

Stauffer (Mayo Clinic): No, I would agree with that treatment regimen.

Treatment done at this stage: We made preoperative judgment that there might be a communication between the bursa and the joint. We opened both the bursa and the joint, and afterwards conducted a synovectomy and debridement of the medial side of the tibia. Inflammatory granulation was observed in the bone, as well. (Fig. 2a). Histological examination revealed septic inflammation invading the bone. However, the prosthesis was not removed because it appeared to be firmly fixed. Two months after debridement, a fistula developed on the medial side of the knee (Fig. 2b). At this stage, what kind of treatment should be performed?

Chairman: What should we do with the second treatment?

Nishioka: If there is no healing after debridement, I think removal must be considered. After removal, bone cement can be used as a spacer.

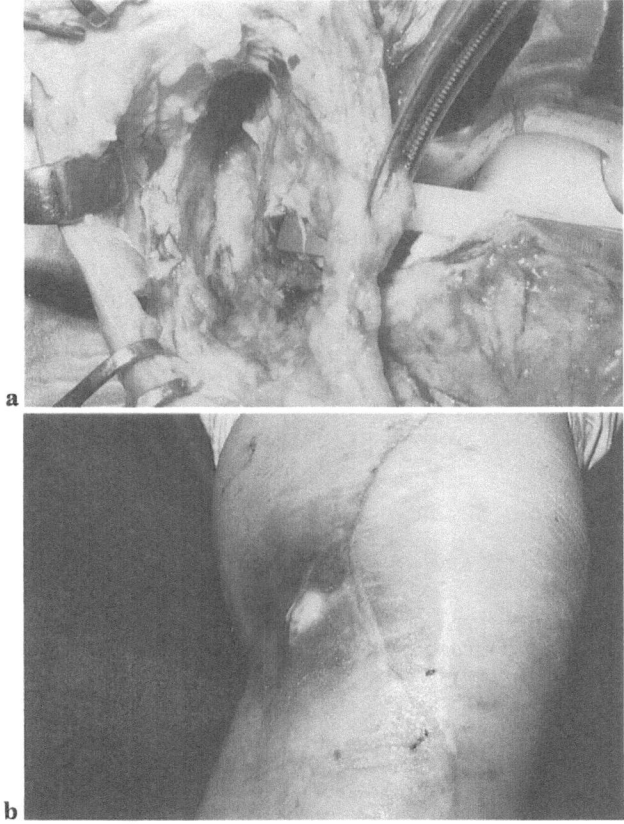

Fig. 2 a At surgery a large inflamed bursa was found communicating with the upper part of the tibia. Histology showed septic bursitis and osteomyelitis. Extensive curettage was done across the entire joint. The tibial prosthesis seemed firmly fixed and was not removed. **b** Two months after curettage a sinus developed on the medial side of the knee

Kawai: Yes, I did. The bone scintigram showed high uptake of 99 m Tc in the medial side of the tibia before and after debridement.

Nishioka (Shiga University): Did you use scintigraphy? What was the development of the lesion?

Chairman: So your opinion is removal. Any other comments from the audience? I think the situation is clear. Most of the audience recommend removal of the implant.

Treatment done at this stage: We removed the prosthesis and performed extensive curettage as suggested. After surgery, the wound healed quickly and there were no clinical symptoms of infection. Fig. 3 shows the anteroposterior and lateral radio-

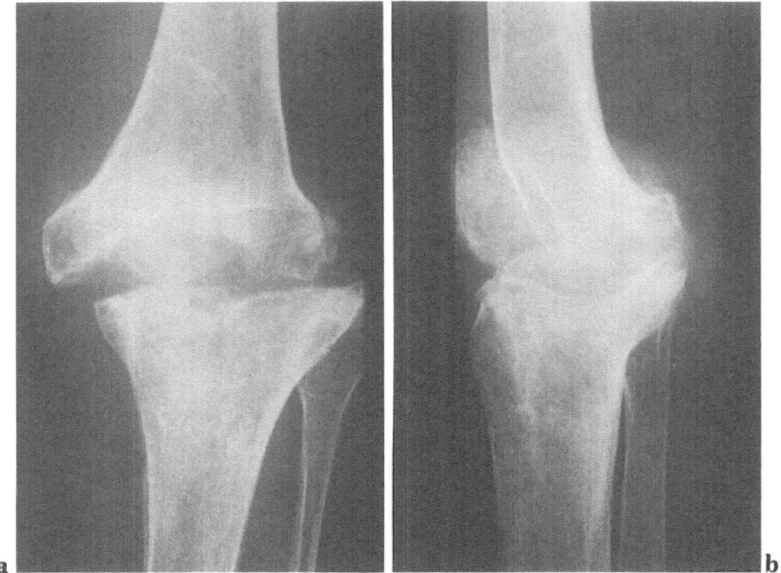

Fig. 3 a,b. X-rays taken 3 months after the removal of the prosthesis show a bone defect of the femur and shortened extensor mechanism. The patella is located close to the tibia

graphs of the knee 3 months after removal of the prosthesis. So, from here, what should be done?

Chairman: Any differing opinions? Dr. Wilde, how would you proceed?

Wilde: At this point, with the wound healed, I would consider reimplantation of another prosthesis. It is interesting that Dr. Filmary at the University of California has reported results on debridement alone in knee infections while leaving the prosthesis in. His series was, I think, about 50 knees, and the treatment was successful in 25% of the cases. So, I think the tendency for us would be, with an established infection (let's say of longer than 2–3 weeks), to just take the prosthesis out.

Chairman: Dr. Stauffer?

Stauffer: I think the only comment I have is that the X-ray here shows what probably would have been the wisdom of Dr. Wilde's suggestion to use an antibiotic-impregnated cement, not only for the local bactericidal effect, but also as a spacer. Now the quadriceps mechanism is shortened and the patella may have even fused to the knee (Fig. 3b). I think now we would certainly try to reimplant it with antibiotic-impregnated cement at this point.

Chairman: Can you give us your current choice of prosthesis? What would you use in this situation?

Stauffer: I think it is the dealer's choice. I would probably use the revision type porous-coated anatomical (PCA), as that is the system that I use. It has a femoral component of differing thicknesses, so you can keep the center of rotation as close to normal as possible. I do cement with an antibiotic.

Wilde: I think you do need a cemented, stemmed prosthesis from the femoral side and also the tibial side, because of the amount of bone lost. One of the major problems will be that it is going to expose the knee, which will be becoming very stiff, and there can be a lot of scars. One way to ease that would be to make a transfer or curved incision through the quadriceps tendon on the lateral side, which would enable you to evert the patella more easily. One of the potential complications in a situation like this, where the exposure is going to be difficult, is going to be avulsion of the infrapatellar tendon. Richard Scott has popularized that particular approach to ease the exposure.

Kawai: I have a question. This is a case of rheumatoid arthritis, so there is no indication or proof that the infection has healed at this point, when 3 months have passed. We have only clinical signs, but there is no proof. At this moment, do you think I could conduct the reimplantation, or do I have to wait for a time? I would like to have your advice, please.

Chairman: So, the exact question is how to determine the status of the knee prior to the implantation.

Wilde: You could aspirate the knee at this point to see if there is any fluid and do a gram-stain and culture. The sedimentation rate may not be too helpful because of the rheumatoid arthritis, but those would be the two things that could be done.

Stauffer: I would add that what I have done is a biopsy of the area, actually using a co-biopsy and taking samples from the adjacent bone as far as aspirating the area without antibiotics, but in the operating room with an image intensifier. I would look at the cultures; and then, if I am satisfied, I would go on.

Chandler (Harvard Medical School): I would agree with Dr. Wilde's suggestion of putting in a methacrylate spacer. As far as exposure, I have no hesitation in taking the tibial tuberosity. We have 33 tibial tuberostomies now in TKR and have only one complication of a fracture through a proximal screw hole. The osteotomy we do is basically what has been described by Triatte for congenital tracking problems. We use a very large segment which should be at least 3–4 in. in length, ½ in. in width, and ¼ in. in thickness. It has to be thick enough that it will not break. We use 2 cancellous screws to fix it and move the knee as if it had not been taken. We have manipulated the knee, put them on bicycles and there is no problem with that.

As far as reconstruction is concerned, I would have a PCA revision component available, but would also have a femoral condyle bone-graft available. We have 37 major knee bone grafts, 3 of them with previous infections. In hips we have 10 patients with previous infections regrafted. Only one of that entire series drained again and that was with the original organism. So, I would lean a little bit more toward reconstructing the bone and particularly the femur, where you can see the anterior portion is gone (Fig. 3b). That can be reconstructed by a slab of femoral condyle, and the tibial defect could be reconstructed with a head and neck. If I could reconstruct easily, I would do that rather than use such a massive component as PCA, although I think that is the best of the revision components. I would tend more toward a resurfacing type of component like PCA tibial component used with cement.

Follow-up: Following this we waited for 1 year. The patient could walk on the external brace with two crutches. An X-ray at that time showed the re-modeled joint surface with marginal sclerosis (Fig. 4). There was no osteolytic sign suggesting infection, but the extensor mechanism was severely shortened. The position of the patella was very low and the patellar ligament was fused to the tibia. The range of motion was also severely limited (flexion 35°, extension 0°). The knee was unstable laterally; while, both bone and soft tissue scintigraphy showed mild and homogeneous uptake of isotope around the knee joint.

Before reimplantation, biopsy specimens from bone and scar tissue were taken and examined histologically. After confirmation of the complete subsidence of the septic inflammation, reimplantation surgery was done using the type of kinematic stabilizer with a long medullary stem, both prostheses being cemented (Fig. 5). An anterior straight incision was made. The knee joint was fibrous and ankylosed (Fig. 6a). Scar tissue was removed extensively and the bone marrow was again debrided. The portion of bone was cut as little as possible with a saw. Then, the trial prosthesis was inserted (thickness of tibial plateau = 8 mm). At this point, the collateral ligament had come into much tension. Therefore, it's insertion and origin were slightly elevated; and lateral release was accomplished by cutting the lateral capsule and tensor facia-latae transversely. Then, the insertion of the patellar tendon was translocated proximally and sutured to the bone. Moreover, the patellar tendon was strengthened with wire (Figs. 5, 6b). The knee achieved a good range of motion (flexion 80°, extension 0°) after these added treatments. On the following day the patient started passive exercise on a continuous passive motion apparatus.

Discussion

Infection is an infrequent but inescapable cause of failure following prosthetic joint replacement. The ratio of deep infection after TKR is higher than that after THR, ranging between 2% and 5% [5–7]. However, appropriate management remains problematic. So far, various kinds of surgical treatment have been reported for infected TKR: (1) synovectomy, (2) removal of the prosthesis, (3) reimplantation, (4) arthrodesis, and (5) amputation. Generally, debridement alone cannot give satisfactory results. Removal of the prosthesis may be necessary in chronic infection [2, 3, 6]. From our experience, only 2 of 11 infected total joint arthroplasty treated primarily by synovectomy had a subsidence of septic inflammation [6]. We now strongly agree with the removal of the prosthesis and extensive curettage for the management of inflected TKR with X-ray abnormalities. After the removal of the prosthesis, arthrodesis of the knee seems most commonly chosen procedure and

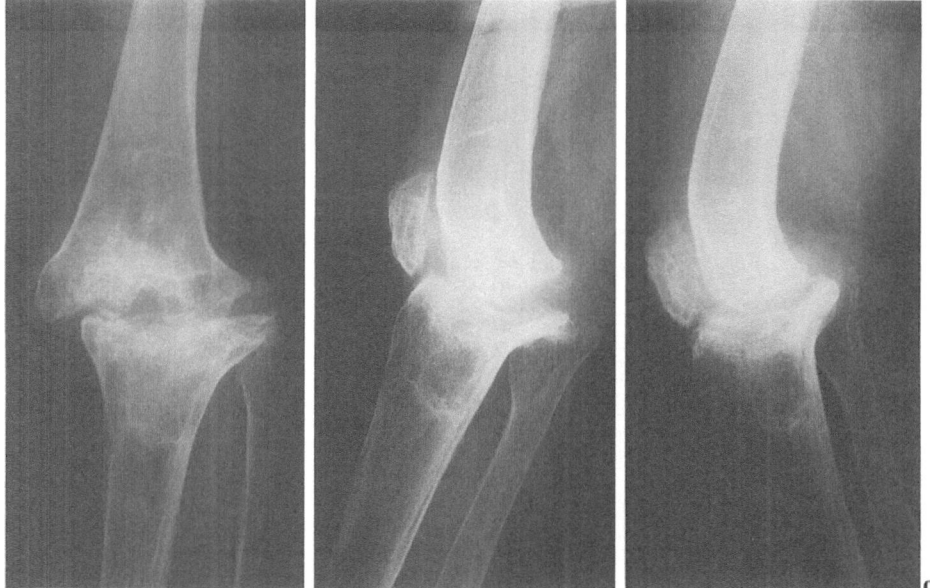

Fig. 4 a-c. X-rays taken a year after the removal of the prosthesis show reconstruction of the new joint with marginal sclerosis. Anteroposterior view (**a**); lateral view in maximum extension (**b**); in maximum flexion (**c**)

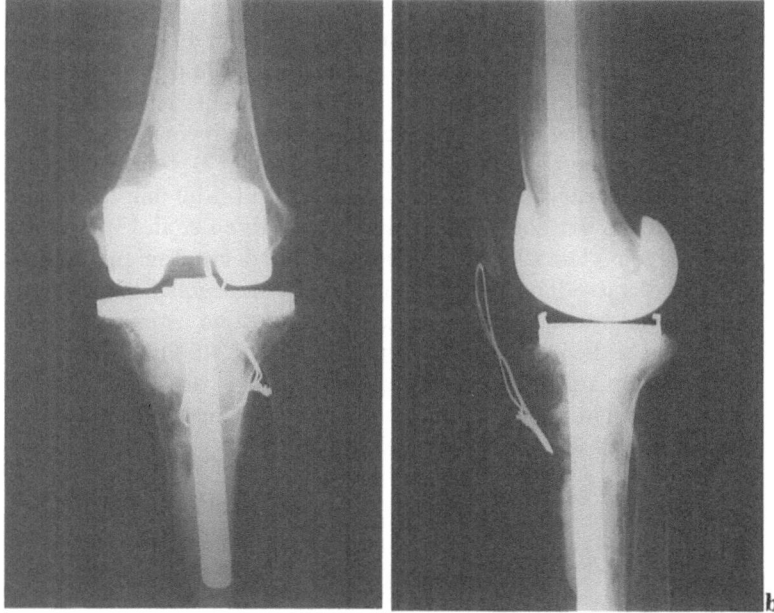

Fig. 5 a,b. X-rays taken 2 weeks after reimplantation. The type of kinematic stabilizer with a long stem was selected as a new prosthesis. Much cement is seen in the medullary canal, but X-rays show good correction of deformity and adequate positioning of the patella

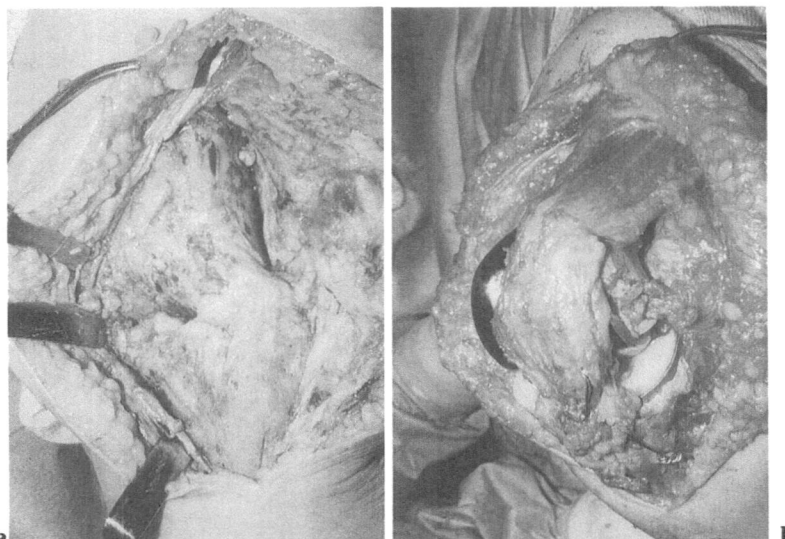

Fig. 6.a Knee joint opened during reimplantation shows joint cavity is replaced by dense collagenous tissue **b** Knee joint just after reimplantation with extensor mechanism reconstructed to raise the patella to its original position. Tensor fascia latae and lateral capsule were cut transversely

satisfactory [2, 5, 7]. On the other hand, reimplantation surgery has become one alternative for maintaining joint motion [3, 4, 7]. In fact, the result of one-stage exchange arthroplasty at the hip was surprisingly improved by using antibiotic-impregnated cement [1]. Since then, revision arthroplasty has met with moderate success and should be employed in certain cases. Freeman et al. [3] reported 8 cases with one-stage revision arthroplasty, and Insall et al. [4], 11 cases with two-stage revision arthroplasty. All of those were successful. Still one-stage reimplantation of a new prosthesis has not yet been established. Rand et al. [7] reported a 63% success rate after reimplantation and mentioned that delayed reimplantaion appeared to be more predictable than early reinsertion of a new prosthesis.

The goals of treatment in our case were infection care and pain relief. If possible, the patient wished to maintain joint motion and stability. Therefore, we performed reimplantaion surgery 1 year after removal. A 3- or 6-month interval before reimplantation might have been better [4, 7], but the reason for the delay was our fear of a recurrence of the infection.

References

1. Bucholz HW, Elson RA, Engelbrecht E, Rottger J, Siegel A, Lodenkamper H (1981) Management of deep infection of total hip replacement. J Bone Joint Surg 63B: 342–353
2. Bliss DG, McBride GG (1985) Infected total knee arthroplasties. Clin Orthop 199: 207–214

3. Freeman MAR, Sudlow RA, Casewell MW, Radcliff SS (1985) The management of in-
    fected total knee replacements. J Bone Joint Surg 67B: 764–768
4. Insall JN, Thompson FM, Brause BD (1983) Two-stage reimplantation for the salvage of
    infected total knee arthroplasty. J Bone Joint Surg 65A: 1087–1098
5. Johnson DP, Bannister GC (1986) The outcome of infected arthroplasty of the knee.
    J Bone Joint Surg 68B: 289–291
6. Kawai K, Shiba R, Hirohata K (1988) Treatment of infected arthroplasty (in Japanese).
    Ryumachi 28 (6): 34–36
7. Rand JA, Bryan RS, Morrey BF, Fred Westholm PA (1986) Management of infected
    total knee arthroplasty. Clin Orthop 205: 75–85

Cup Arthroplasty in a 31-Year-Old Female with Neglected Congenital Dislocation of the Hip

RYOICHI SHIBA[1]

Summary. Cup arthroplasty combined with Chiari's osteotomy was performed on a 31-year-old female with neglected congenital dislocation of the left hip. The 11-year follow-up examination is reported here.

Case Presentation

Present illness. The patient is a 31-year-old female who is married but does not have any children. Her chief complaint was pain of the left hip and limping.

At 2 years old, as initial walking was quite delayed, she was found to have congenital dislocation of the left hip. At that time, open reduction was performed. From that time until up to 30 years of age she did not have any pain and could enjoy sports. At the age of 30, she began to have pain during walking and after walking. She also began limping. Her symptoms gradually conspicuous, and thus, she came to Kobe University Hospital at the age of 31 years for consultation.

Present status. Upon examination, the Trendelenburg sign was positive. There was flexion of the hip joint of 130°, extension 0°, abduction 30°, adduction 20°, internal rotation 40°, and external rotation 45°. Leg length discrepancy was 3 cm. According to the Japanese Orthopedics Association (JOA) hip evaluation, her pain score was 20 points (full mark, 40 points), walking ability, 15 points (out of 20), range of motion (ROM), 15 points (out of 20), activities of daily living, 17 points (out of 20) and her total score was 72 points out of 100 points.

Roentgenogram. The roentgenogram findings (Fig. 1) showed a dislocation of the left hip joint. The neck shaft angle was 135°, and antetorsion was 10°. The primary acetabulum was dysplastic and the femoral head was in contact with the secondary acetabulum. When the left leg was pulled down, the femoral head came closer to the primary acetabulum. However, it could not be reduced in the primary acetabulum. Better congruity was not achievable by abduction or adduction. The arthrogram indicated cartilagenous coverage on the surface of both the femoral head and acetabulum.

---

[1] Department of Orthopedic Surgery, Kobe University School of Medicine, Kobe, Japan

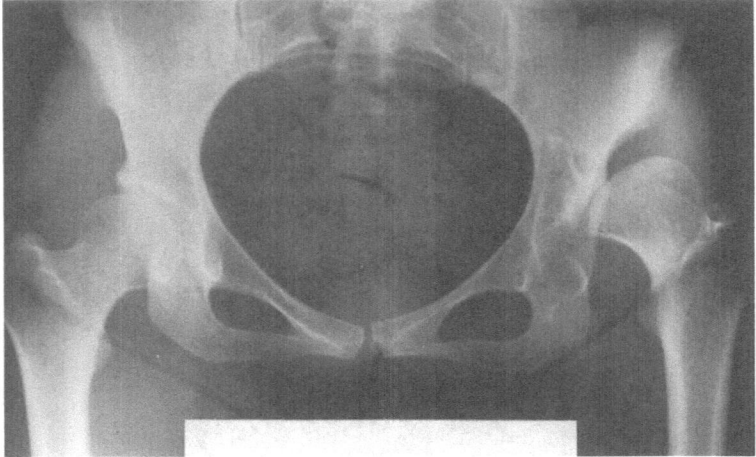

Fig. 1. Roentgenogram before operation

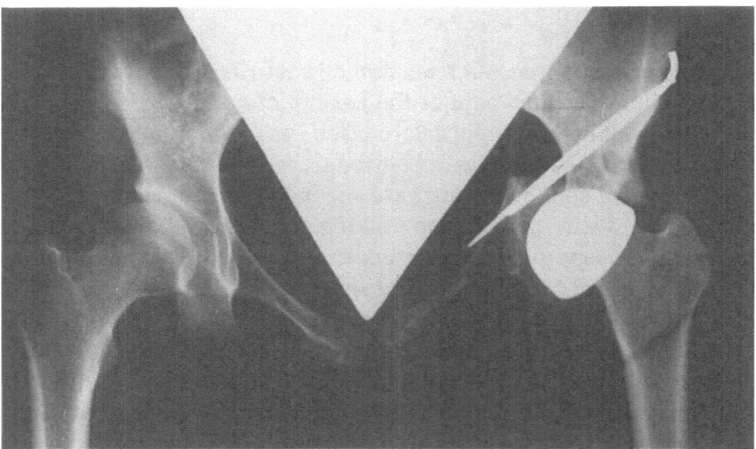

Fig. 2. Roentgenogram immediately after the operation

Treatment

Procedure. Cup arthroplasty combined with Chiari's pelvic osteotomy was performed without preoperative traction (Fig. 2).

Postoperative treatment. Isometric muscle exercise was started from the 2nd day after the operation, ROM exercise and muscle training from the 3rd week, partial weight bearing from the 9th week, and full weight bearing without crutches or a cane from the 7th month.

Follow-up

At the 11-year follow-up, the Trendelenburg sign was negative and the patient did not limp (Fig. 3). The leg length discrepancy was 0.5 cm, with flexion 110°, extension 0°, abduction 30°, adduction 18°, internal rotation 30°, and external rotation 30°. The JOA score was 100 points. She could walk without a cane for more than 60 min, and could enjoy her life without any limitations (Figs. 4–7). The roentgenogram findings (Fig. 8) showed good congruity, and excellent positioning of the cup. A radiolucent line, which indicates the thickness of the fibrocartilage, can be seen in-between the remolded acetabulum and the cup.

Fig. 3. Negative Trendelenburg sign (at 11-year follow-up exam)

Fig. 4. Japanese-style sitting (at follow-up)

Fig. 5. Japanese-style bowing (at follow-up)

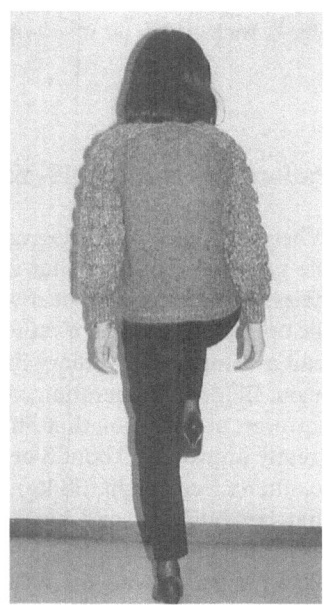

Fig. 3

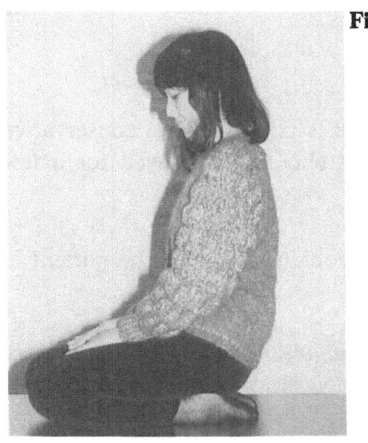

Fig. 4

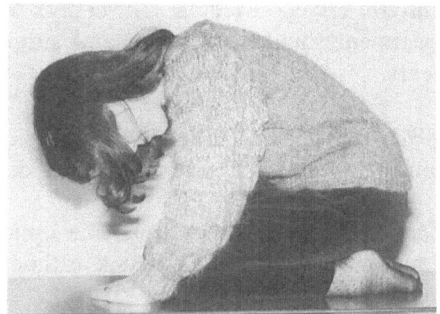

Fig. 5

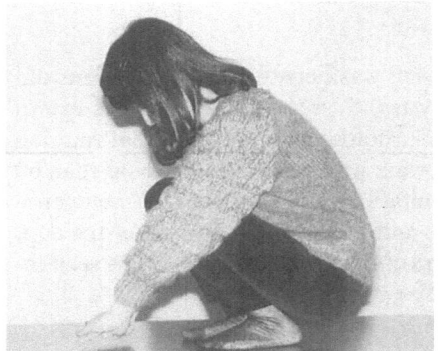

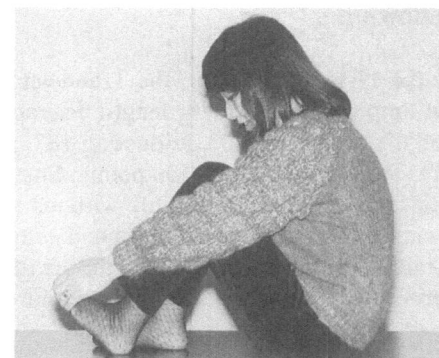

Fig. 6   Fig. 7

Fig. 6. Squatting (at follow-up)

Fig. 7. Nail cutting (at follow-up)

Patient Interview at 11-Year Postoperative Follow-up

When asked about the degree of pain before the operation, the patient revealed that the pain was so severe that she could not walk, and she particularly could not use stairs. She dragged her feet when walking. Regarding the amount of pain following the operation, she had a rather strange sensation in her left hip only. She was able to lead a completely ordinary lifestyle without paying attention to her feet after 3 or 4 years. Before the operation, the lower limb was shorter by 3 cm, causing her to limp; however, at operation that difference was improved to 0.5 cm, and thus her limp was greatly improved. About 3 or 4 years after the operation the limp was not noticeable to others. Her weight (38 kg) is the same now as it was before the operation. She said that her husband and parents were helpful in assisting her rehabilitation. When asked her overall impression concerning the surgery, she said that she was completely satisfied with the results.

Discussion

Tateishi (Hyogo Medical University): When the pain is not so severe, conservative treatment should be chosen and surgical treatment should be delayed for a few years.

Wilde (Cleveland Clinic): It is a very challenging problem, because the patient is young and obviously has progressive disability.

Cooke (Queen's University): The options of surgical treatment are actually very limited, because it does not look as though any kind of varus or valgus femoral osteotomies would provide cover.

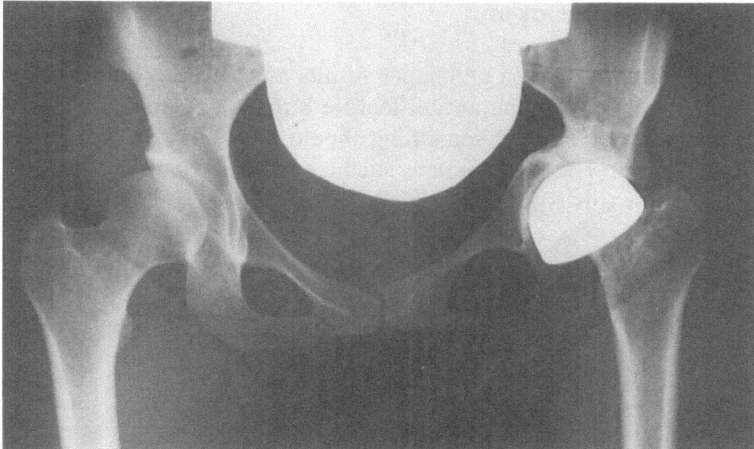

Fig. 8. Roentgenográm at 11-year follow-up

Tanaka (Kinki University): Since there was cartilage on the surface of the femoral head, the shelf operation is indicated after a period of skeletal traction prior to the surgery.

Huang (Beijing): For this type of neglected congenital dislocation of the hip (CDH), Chiari's pelvic osteotomy is indicated if the femoral head can pulled down with 4 weeks of skeletal traction. If the femoral head is rigid, femoral osteotomy has to be combined.

Chandler (Harvard Medical School): I would lean more toward the Chiari's osteotomy. Chiari's osteotomy is a conservative operation; it does not burn any bridges. It is not going to give her a perfect hip. She would have to realize that it is the first stage, and the later stage would be uncemented total hip replacement. However, if she could wait until better devices were available, that would be the best.

Stauffer (Mayo Clinic): To do Chiari's osteotomy and obtain coverage of the femoral head however, you have to displace it completely. I wonder if that is possible? So a porous-coated hip replacement could be indicated even in a 31-year-old.

Wilde: Chiari's osteotomy would be the choice here. We are beginning to see more of the problems of the porous-coated devices.

Cooke: Whether Chiari's osteotomy would be successful or not is a dilema, because Chiari's ostoetomy, with this degree of subluxation puts too much pressure on the femoral head and not enough coverage or support. So, the options might be to consider fusion or to consider some kind of special reconstruction of the hip.

Wilde: This is a 31-year-old woman who is sexually active and in the child-bearing years. Hip fusion is not a good choice for such a woman.

Chairman's Conclusion

Cooke: I think this case had super results and no one could possibly look for any better. I feel the really important feature is that this result gives her a tremendously acetabular base. Thus, if something should happen in the future, reconstruction is so much easier, because you have such a good base to work with. I think that is the real place for this type of treatment.

Postscript

The 10th anniversary of a professorship is a very special event, and what better way to celebrate it than to host a conference? In the Department of Orthopedic Surgery at Kobe University Medical School, this special event was in honor of Kazushi Hirohata, the second professor of orthopaedics at this school. A most appropriate feature of the conference was its international flavor — guests came from Germany, Canada, and the United States. It is noteworthy that this international flavor reflects the commitment of Kazushi Hirohata's professorship, since he has now many research and clinical fellows who have spent time in American, Canadian, and European centers. It is important also to know that the breadth of their, and thereby Kobe's, orientation in orthopedics is increasingly wide; it has always had a very strong thrust in arthritis and rheumatic disease research.

This conference focused on joint reconstruction, not just the usual themes, but the problem areas with new basic science approaches as well as new clinical techniques. For those clinicians still eager to learn from case reports, there were excellent examples here for us to enjoy.

For those of us who know Professor Hirohata and his colleagues in this excellent school, the conference was, as usual, high caliber, beautifully organized, and wonderfully hosted. To have taken part was an honor and a great pleasure for which I extend, on behalf of all the guests from abroad, our heartfelt appreciation.

For me, this volume is also special as I had an opportunity to edit and work with the material during my visiting professorship to Kobe, during the spring of 1988, the first in orthopedics to be sponsored by the Japanese government. It was an unforgettably happy and enriching experience. Thank you Kobe University, Department of Orthopedics, thank you Kazushi, and your team.

T. DEREK V. COOKE
Joint Surgery
Visiting Professor
Kobe University

Subject Index

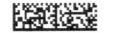